AF820829

Clinical Implications of Irritable Bowel Syndrome

Edited by
Philippe Denis

Walter de Gruyter
Berlin · New York 1997

Editor

Prof. Dr. P. Denis
Groupe de Biochemie et de Physiopathologie Digestive et Nutritionelle (GBPDN)
CHU Rouen
F-76031 Rouen Cedex
France

Produced with an educational grant of Solvay Pharmaceuticals, Hannover, Germany.

Deutsche Bibliothek – Cataloging-in-Publication-Data

Clinical implications of irritable bowel syndrome / ed. by Philippe Denis. – Berlin ; New York : de Gruyter, 1997
ISBN 3-11-015860-4

© Copyright 1997 by Walter de Gruyter & Co., Berlin. All rights reserved, including those of translation into foreign languages. No part of this book may be reproduced in any form – by photoprint, microfilm or any other means nor transmitted nor translated into a machine language without written permission from the publisher.

Medical science is constantly developing. Research and clinical experience expand our knowledge, especially with regard to treatment and medication.

For dosages and applications mentioned in this work, the reader may rely on the authors, editors and publisher having taken great pains to ensure that these indications reflect the standard of knowledge at the time this work was completed.

Nevertheless, all users are requested to check the package leaflet of the medication, in order to determine for themselves whether the recommendations given for the dosages or the likely contraindications differ from those given in this book. This is especially true for medication which is seldom used or has recently been put on the market and for medication whose application has been restricted by the German Ministry of Health.

The quotation of registered names, trade names, trade marks, etc. in this copy does not imply, even in the absence of a specific statement that such names are exempt from laws and regulations protecting trade marks, etc. and therefore free for general use.

Typesetting and Printing: Arthur Collignon GmbH, Berlin. – Binding: Lüderitz & Bauer, Berlin. – Printed in Germany.

Authors

H. Bosseckert, Prof. Dr.
Friedrich-Schiller-Universität Jena
Klinikum für Innere Medizin
D-00740 Jena
Germany

M. Delvaux, Dr.
Gastroenterology Unit
CHU Rangueil
F-31054 Toulouse
France

P. Denis, Prof. Dr.
Groupe de Biochémie et de
Physiopathologie Digestive et
Nutritionelle (GBPDN)
DHU Rouen
F-76031 Rouen Cedex
France

C. P. Fletcher, Dr.
Thornham House
Ermington
Nr. Ivybridge
South Devon PL 21 OLG
United Kingdom

P. Guyot, Dr.
5, avenue Jean Jaurès
F-69077 Lyon
France

W. E. Whitehead, Prof. Dr.
Division of Digestive Disease & Nutrition
Department of Medicine
CB# 7080, Room 326
Burnett-Womack building
University of North Carolina at
Chapel Hill
Chapel Hill, N.C. 27599-7080
USA

Contents

Introduction

P. Denis

Functional gastrointestinal disorders especially irritable bowel syndrome (IBS) is currently gaining in importance in the field of gastroenterology during the last years.

It was the aim of this round table organised by Solvay Pharmaceuticals to give an overview of the most interesting developments in IBS.

The psychosocial aspects of functional gastrointestinal disorders were discussed by W. E. Whitehead. The indepth analysis of the patients' behaviour, the knowledge about the influence of childhood social learning and traumatic events, as well as the role of psychosocial factors have changed the unterstanding of IBS. However, although they seem to be comorbid conditions, they do not cause IBS but influence the patient's decision to consult a physician.

Abdominal pain is the cardinal symptom of IBS and the backbone of the diagnosis as explained by H. Bosseckert. But this symptom is the most problematic, too, because it is present in other severe gastrointestinal disorders. An overview is given where the pitfalls of diagnosis are and how reliable the available criteria are.

Visceral hypersensitivity is one of the most promising approaches to the pathophysiology of IBS. The knowledge about the so-called gut-brain axis and the enteric nervous system has increased tremendously. M. Delvaux refers to the clinical relevance and shows a way through the jungle.

In the last part of this round table two new studies on mebeverine slow release formulation were presented.

First, the new drug was compared to the plain mebeverine formulation under very strict IBS inclusion criteria and an up-to-date IBS evaluation design for the symptoms. The results are presented by one of the investigators of this study, C. P. Fletcher.

The aim of the other study was to identify special IBS symptom subgroups more sensitive to the mebeverine slow release treatment. P. Guyot shows whether the treatmant window for mebeverine is smaller or broader.

Psychosocial aspects of functional gastrointestinal disorders

W. E. Whitehead

Introduction

The aims of this presentation are (a) to describe the types of psychiatric disorders and psychological traits found in patients with functional gastrointestinal disorders (GI) disorders, with special attention to (b) the question of whether irritable bowel syndrome is a somatization disorder; (c) to discuss whether irritable bowel syndrome (IBS) and functional dyspepsia are distinct disorders based on factor analysis of gastrointestinal symptoms in large groups of subjects; and to describe (d) the role of psychosocial stress and sexual abuse and (e) the role of childhood reinforcement and modelling in the etiology and course of IBS. The paper will conclude with (f) a model of how psychological factors interact with physiological factors to influence the expression of functional GI disorders.

Psychiatric disorders in IBS

Five studies (tab. 1) have assessed the prevalence of psychiatric disorders in patients with irritable bowel syndrome using standardized interviews or the Diagnostic Interview Schedule administered by trained lay interviewers [1]. From 42% to 93% of patients with functional bowel disorders meet criteria for a psychiatric diagnosis compared to a median incidence of 19% in patients

Table 1 Prevalence of psychiatric disorders in IBS

Source	N	IBS	ORGANIC	CONTROL
Ford et al. (1987)	44	42%	6%	8%
Corney et al. (1990)	48	48%	–	–
Toner et al. (1990)	44	61%	–	14%
Blanchard (1990)	68	56%	25%	18%
Walker et al. (1990)	28	93%	19%	–
Aggregate	232	57%	–	–

Adapted from Reference [1].

with organic gastrointestinal disorders and 14% in healthy controls. The most common diagnosis is depression [2] and antidepressant medications are coming to be recognized as particularly effective for the treatment of IBS [3]. However, no diagnosis is uniquely associated with IBS.

The incidence of anxiety disorders is high in IBS, and Lydiard and colleagues [4] have suggested that panic disorder is one cause of IBS. However, subsequent studies have shown that relatively few patients with panic attacks meet criteria for IBS, and relatively few patients with IBS admit to panic attacks [5–6]. This suggests that the association between IBS and panic attacks may be a spurious one which is due either to the tendency for patients with panic attacks to report multiple somatic symptoms or to the tendency for high levels of anxiety to cause diarrhea and abdominal pain.

Psychological traits

Psychological tests completed by patients with IBS show levels and types of psychopathology similar to what is revealed by psychiatric diagnostic interviews: IBS patients and patients with a nonspecific functional bowel disorder show elevations on the Beck Depression Inventory and the Spielberger State-Trait Anxiety Inventory [2]. On the Pilowsky [2] Illness Behavior Inventory (fig. 1), IBS patients show significant elevations on the scales for Disease Phobia and Disease Conviction (scales which define hypochondriasis), and on scales

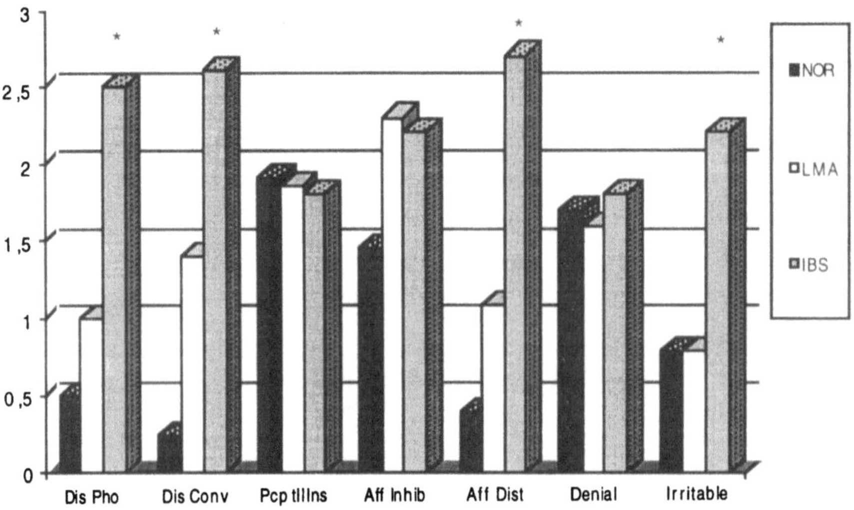

Fig. 1 Illness behavior questionnaire (Adapted from Reference [2]).

for Affective Disturbance and Irritability (scales which are related to depression and anxiety). IBS patients also show elevations on tests measuring general psychological distress [7–8] and on personality tests measuring neuroticism [9].

Somatization disorder

Somatization refers to a tendency for a subgroup of anxious and depressed patients to report multiple somatic symptoms without objective evidence of disease, as the primary manifestation of their psychological distress. Some have argued that IBS is a somatization disorder [9–10] rather than a motility disorder or a disorder of visceral perception, and there is data to support this, as summarized below:

IBS patients report more non-gastrointestinal symptoms (fig. 2) than the general population [11–12]: There is an excess incidence of fibromyalgia [13–14], dysmenorrhea [15–16], detrusor instability [17], and other non-colonic symptoms or disorders [18]. It has even been suggested that the presence of these nongastrointestinal symptoms is common enough to provide a diagnostic marker for IBS [18].

Disability days [11, 19] and clinic visits [11] (fig. 3) for non-gastrointestinal symptoms are also elevated in patients with IBS compared to the rest of the

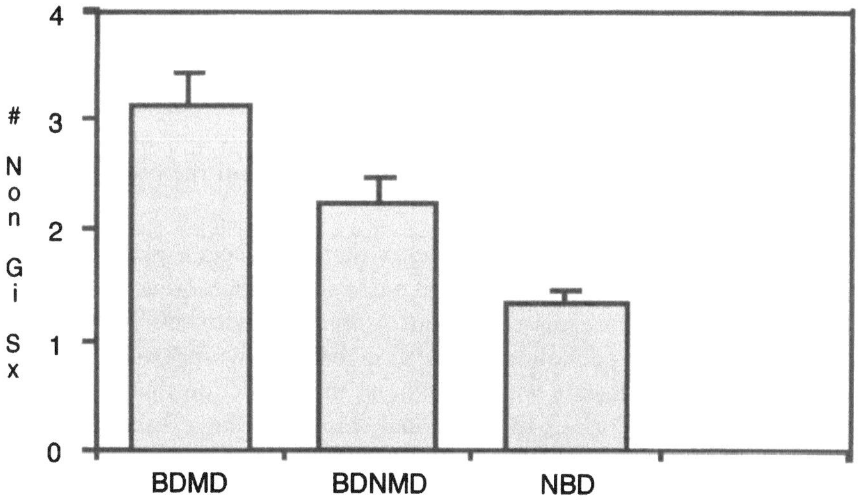

Fig. 2 Multiple somatic complaints in patients with IBS. BDMD refers to patients with a functional bowel disorder who have consulted a physician; BDNMD refers to patients with a functional bowel disorder who have *not* consulted a physician; and NBD refers to people without a functional bowel disorder (Adapted from Reference [11].

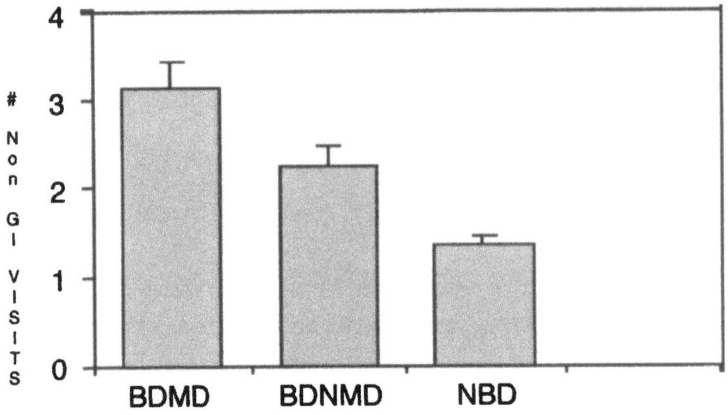

Fig. 3 Multiple doctor visits in patients with IBS. BDMD refers to patients with a functional bowel disorder who have consulted a physician; BDNMD refers to patients with a functional bowel disorder who have *not* consulted a physician; and NBD refers to people without a functional bowel disorder (Adapted from Reference [11]).

population, and patients with IBS undergo more surgical procedures, especially hysterectomies (in women)[20, 21]. The outpatient health care costs of IBS patients are approximately twice as much as the outpatient health care costs of the rest of the population.

The mechanisms responsible for somatiozation are not well understood. It has been suggested that anxiety can lower the threshold for labeling as painful or as a symptom of disease, the somatic sensations caused by normal physiological events [22]. Consistent with this hypothesis, the physiological events associated with IBS (i. e., segmental contractions of the colon [23], discrete clustered contractions [24] and giant ileal contractions of the small intestine [25], and altered thresholds for perception of intraluminal distention [26] are not qualitatively different, although they may be quantitatively different from the physiological activity seen in healthy controls [9, 27].

An alternative explanation for somatization is that it reflects a psychological tendency to attribute disease significance to sensations which other people ignore or treat as normal (i. e., misattribution). Consistent with this hypothesis, studies of patients with hypochondriasis suggest that the two principal dimensions of this disorder are disease conviction (i. e., the conviction that one has a disease) and disease phobia (i. e., the irrational fear of having a disease) [28].

The somatization hypothesis to explain IBS is plausible for the reasons described above and because there are no physiological markers for IBS. However, two types of evidence suggest that more than somatization is involved in the etiology of IBS: First, a large number of people meet diaxgnostic criteria for IBS but have no evidence of psychopathology [7, 29] and no tendency to report other disorders. Only 20–40% of people who meet symptom criteria consult physicians for these symptoms [7, 19]. Secondly, factor analysis of GI symptoms in large populations shows that these symptoms cluster together in patterns which are consistent with IBS and other functional GI disorders [30, 31]. One would not expect specific symptom clusters if a generalized tendency to report somatic symptoms led to the diagnosis of these disorders.

Are IBS and functional dyspepsia different disorders?

An important special case of the somatization hypothesis is the question of whether IBS and functional dyspepsia are different disorders or part of the same disorder. These two functional gastrointestinal disorders share many common features: (a) Pain is the cardinal symptom of both. (b) Visceral hyperalgesia as demonstrated by a reduced threshold to report pain from distention of the lumen of the bowel, characterizes both disorders. Some studies suggest that visceral hyperalgesia occurs throughout the gastrointestinal tract such that patients with IBS have a lower threshold for distention of the stomach as well as the lower bowel, and patients with functional dyspepsia have a lower threshold for distention of the rectum as well as the stomach and esophagus [32]. (c) Depending on the diagnostic criteria used, there may be a substantial overlap in the diagnosis of IBS and dyspepsia: For example, we found in a population-based survey of U.S. adults (tab. 2) that when functional dyspepsia was defined only as upper abdominal pain or discomfort [33], 28.4% of people with functional dyspepsia also met criteria for IBS (compared to a population prevalence of IBS of 11.6%). Data such as these have led some to conclude that IBS and dyspepsia (and perhaps other functional gastrointestinal disorders as well) are different aspects of the same disorder [34]. However, there are two types of evidence which argue for the relative independence of IBS and functional dyspepsia.

Table 2 Overlap among diagnoses – U. S. householder survey of 5,340

	IBS	F.I.	Proct	Dysch
Dyspep	28.4	--	--	--
IBS	--	21.1	34.3	42.4
Constip	--	12.2	23.4	96.5
Incontin	30.2	--	27.6	26.2
Proctalg	33.1	18.6	--	37.0
Dyschez	38.9	16.8	35.3	--
Preval	11.6	7.8	11.6	13.8

First, factor analysis of bowel symptoms in large groups of normal subjects [33] and medical patients [35] identifies discrete clusters of symptoms corresponding to IBS, ulcer-like dyspepsia, and dysmotility-like dyspepsia. If these were different aspects of the same disorder, one would not expect separate factors to emerge.

Second, there is less overlap in diagnoses made by the Rome criteria than at first appears. The recommendation of the Rome committee that functional dyspepsia be made on the basis of upper GI pain or discomfort alone cannot be accepted because more than half of unselected patients attending a medical clinic endorse this symptom [35]. Rather, the diagnosis of functional dyspepsia should be restricted to the subtypes, ulcer-like and dysmotility-like dyspepsia as defined by the Rome committee [36], for which there is support from factor analysis studies [33, 35]. When this is done, the overlap between IBS and either ulcer-like or dysmotility-like dyspepsia is no greater than would be expected by change. It is also interesting to note that in neither Talley's data [37] nor in our data [33, 35] is the overlap between ulcer-like and dysmotility-like dyspepsia very great: Rather they form separate clusters of symptoms.

Self-selection for treatment

There is evidence to suggest that psychological symptoms/disorders do not cause IBS but, when psychological symptoms coexist with IBS, they may influence the patient's decision to seek treatment. The evidence for this hypothesis is that people with IBS who have not consulted a physician are no more psychologically distressed than the rest of the population, although patients with IBS who are seen in medical clinics are usually found to be psychologically distressed, and a high proportion of them have a coexisting psychiatric disorder [7, 38, 39]. This suggests that the high incidence of psychological abnormalities seen in medical clinics may be an artifact of self-selection for treatment by psychologically distressed individuals.

Role of psychological stress

A majority of patients with IBS and nearly half of the people without IBS report that psychological stress triggers abdominal pain and/or diarrhea [40]. This association is supported by most [40], although not by all [41] studies which have used standardized scales of stressful life events.

One of the more carefully done studies [40] assessed life event stress and bowel symptoms in 383 young women at three-months intervals for one year (fig. 4).

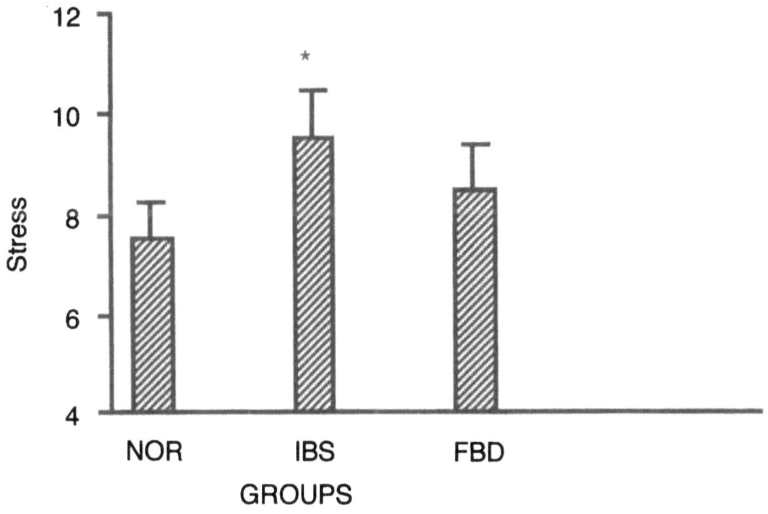

Fig. 4 NOR refers to healthy control women; IBS refers to women meeting restrictive criteria similar to the Rome criteria for irritable bowel syndrome; and FBD refers to women with a nonspecific functional bowel disorder (Adapted from Reference [40]).

The confounding effects of neuroticism were statistically controlled. This study found that stress could explain about 10% of the variance in bowel symptoms, which is both statistically and clinically significant but less than one percent would predict from the frequency with which people attribute their bowel symptoms to stress. This suggests that people exaggerate the importance of stress in an effort after meaning (i. e., a tendency to dismiss inexplicable events and to focus on those which seem to have a recognizable cause). The investigators also demonstrated that stressful life events had a greater impact on the bowel symptoms of women with IBS than they did for women without chronic bowel symptoms. This is consistent with experimental data suggesting that IBS patients show a greater change in colonic motility in response to provocative events than do people without IBS [23].

Studies using standardized life-events scales [40] or structured interviews to measure stress have generally failed to identify specific types of current stressors that are uniquely associated with IBS. The recent stressors most frequently identified by IBS patients as triggers for their symptoms are commonplace worries about relationships, finances, and career [42], or worries about the occurrence of the symptoms [43]. However, there is now a large body of evidence showing that two types of (recalled) childhood traumatic events are significantly more likely to be reported by IBS patients than by control subjects. These are (a) separations from one or both parents by death or marital dissolution during childhood [44–46], and (b) a history of sexual and physical abuse (see below).

Sexual abuse in IBS

The association between sexual abuse and IBS is striking, with more than a third of women with IBS seen in academic medical centers reporting abuse [47]. This observation has now been replicated in a variety of settings including community surveys [48] and primary care clinics [12]. The prevalence of sexual and physical abuse in women with IBS is less in the community and in primary care, but it is still greater than is seen in women without IBS. Possible explanations for this relationship are discussed in a working team report by Drossman and colleagues [49]. It appears that abuse does not cause IBS but that, like neuroticism and psychological distress, it influences which patients seek medical care for their bowel symptoms through self-selection for treatment. The evidence favoring this interpretation is that, at least in academic medical centers, patients with organic disease also have a higher than expected incidence of self-reported sexual abuse even though the incidence is lower than that seen in functional gastrointestinal disorders [47].

Childhood social learning

In a series of studies, my laboratory has investigated the role of childhood learning on the development of IBS and other functional disorders. In the first study [50], we telephone 864 adults in metropolitan Cincinnati and asked them what symptoms they had currently, how they coped with cold or influenza symptoms (e. g., by consulting a physician and staying home from work vs. carrying on with usual activities), and how their parents had responded to them when they had cold or flu symptoms during their childhood. Patients with a functional bowel disorder (abdominal pain and altered bowel habits) were more likely than controls to report that when they were sick as children, their parents gave them gifts and special privileges. We inferred that these gifts and privileges acted as reinforcers of illness behavior and lead to an enduring tendency to notice and report more somatic symptoms. Another laboratory made similar observations [46].

In the next study [51], which dealt with dysmenorrhea and other menstrual symptoms rather than with IBS, we investigated the specificity of childhood social learning: We developed separate scales to measure reinforcement and modeling of menstrual symptoms and cold symptoms, and gave these scales to nursing students and to their mothers. We extended our earlier findings by showing (a) that childhood social learning affects disability days as well as symptom reports, and (b) that childhood learning is relatively specific in that adults complain of the same symptoms which their parents reinforced when they were children.

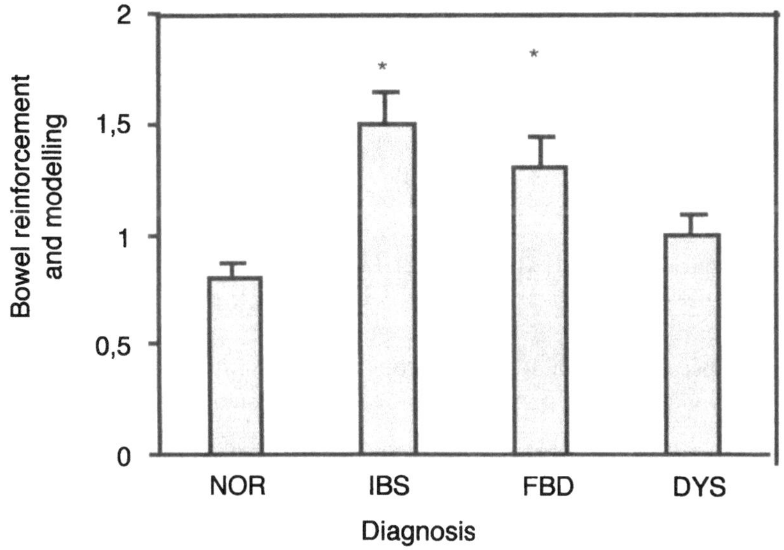

Fig. 5 NOR refers to healthy control women; IBS refers to women meeting restrictive criteria similar to the Rome criteria for irritable bowel syndrome; FBD refers to women with a nonspecific functional bowel disorder; and DYS refers to women with dysmenorrhea. The hypothesis tested in this study is that specific forms of illness behavior are learned during childhood. This graph shows that women with IBS and FBD reports significantly more reinforcement and modeling of bowel-related illness behavior during childhood but women with dysmenorrhea do not. Conversely, women with dysmenorrhea scored higher than the NOR group on a scale measuring childhood reinforcement and modeling of menstrual-related illness behavior (Adapted from Reference [52]).

In our most recent study on this topic [52], we again addressed the issue of specificity of learning by developing scales for the reinforcement and modeling of bowel symptoms during childhood which we could administer along with the scales for reinforcement and modeling of cold and menstrual symptoms. This permitted us to reassess the specificity of learning (fig. 5). An additional feature of this study was that we tested for neuroticism, psychological stress, and physical examination findings in order to see whether the effects of reinforcement and modeling could be shown when these other influences on symptom reporting were held constant by statistical adjustment. This study replicated our earlier observation that adults tend to report the same symptoms that their parents reinforced during childhood, and we showed for the first time that the effects of reinforcement and modeling were independent of the effects of stress and neuroticism. We are currently analyzing the data from a large health maintenance organization which further supports these (previously retrospective) observations by showing that the children of parents who consult a physician for IBS have significantly more visits for abdominal pain and diarrhea than control children even after statistically controlling for the overall utilization of health care by their parents. Thus, it appears that childhood social learning contributes to the development of IBS and possibly to other gastrointestinal motility disorders as well.

How do psychosocial factors and physiological factors interact?

Figure 6 is a schematic of how psychological factors may interact with contractile activity in the small and large intestines, and with pain threshold to affect the perception of IBS symptoms and the patient's decision to act on them by consulting a physician. The majority of patients with IBS have a low threshold to report pain when a balloon is distended in the lumen of the bowel, but balloon distention is a non-physiological stimulus – it is meant to mimic intraluminal distention which may occur as the direct result of intestinal contractions or as the indirect result of nonperistaltic contractions which cause a functional obstruction with distention proximal to the obstruction.

Psychological factors might affect this process at two points: (a) Psychological stress is known to stimulate increased contractile activity in the intestine [23, 24]. We believe, however, that (b) the more important effect is the influence of psychological distress and neuroticism on the threshold at which people notice their gastrointestinal sensations and interpret them as symptoms of disease.

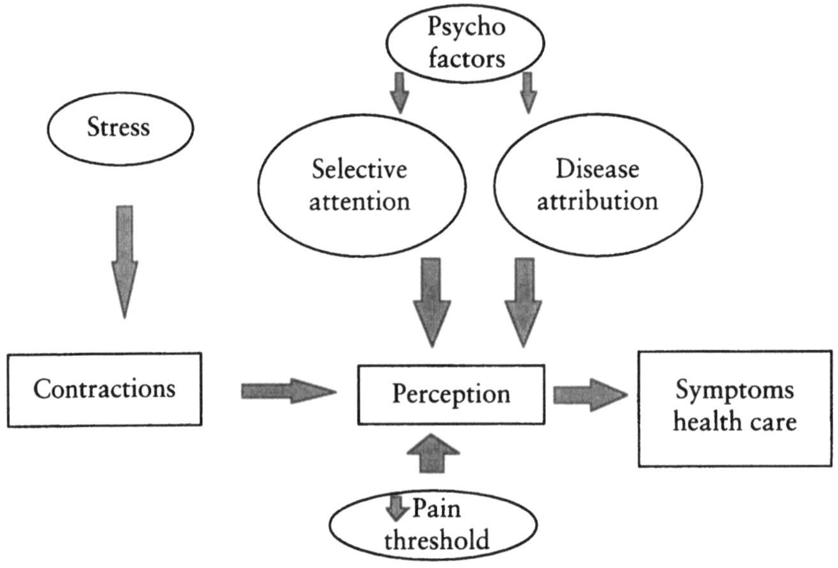

Fig. 6 Model showing possible interactions between psychological factors and physiological mechanisms for the symptoms of IBS. See text for explanation.

We suggest that the effects of neuroticism and psychological distress on pain perception act through two psychological mechanisms: selective attention to gastrointestinal sensations and a tendency to interpret these sensations as symptoms of disease. These two psychological mechanisms are distinct but are related to each other in a positive feedback loop such that a strong tendency to interpret gastrointestinal sensations as symptoms of disease leads to increased vigilance in attending to these sensations, and increased attention leads to the perception of more gastrointestinal sensations which increase the conviction that one may have a disease.

Conclusions

Psychological symptoms (and psychiatric disorders) are common in patients with IBS who are seen in medical centers, but the majority of people with IBS do not consult physicians and are no more psychologically distressed than the rest of the population. These psychiatric disorders are believed to be comorbid conditions which do not cause IBS but which do influence the patient's decision to consult a physician.

Patients with IBS report experiencing more stressful life events, and IBS patients appear to show a greater increase in gastrointestinal symptoms when exposed to stressors. The recent stressors which IBS patients identify as triggering their symptoms are not unique to IBS but are everyday worries about relationships, finances, and career advancement. However, two types of childhood stressors are more common in IBS patients: early separation from parents and sexual and physical abuse. These early trauma probably do not cause IBS but instead influence which patients consult physicians for management of their bowel symptoms.

A characteristic of many patients who consult gastroenterologists for IBS and other motility disorders is a tendency to report multiple somatic complaints (including many non-gastrointestinal complaints) and to over-utilize medical resources. This pattern of behavior is referred to as somatization or abnormal illness behavior. One source of abnormal illness behavior is childhood social learning which occurs (a) when parents provide gifts or special privileges to a child who reports somatic symptoms or (b) when parents model abnormal illness behaviors themselves.

References

[1] Drossman, D. A., Creed, F. H., Fava, G. A., Olden, K. W., Patrick, D. L., Toner, B. B., Whitehead, W. E.: Psychosocial aspects of the functional gastrointestinal disorders. Gastroenterol Int 1995, 8: 47–90.

[2] Whitehead, W. E., Enck, P., Anthony, J. C. , Schuster, M. M.: Psychopathology in patients with irritable bowel syndrome. In: Singer, M. V., Goebell, H. (eds.), Nerves and the gastrointestinal tract. New York, Academic Press 1989, 465–476.
[3] Greenbaum, D. S., Mayle, J. E., Vanegeren, L. E. et al.: Effects of desipramine on irritable bowel syndrome compared with atropine and placebo. Dig Dis Sci 1987, 32: 257–266.
[4] Lydiard, R. B., Laraia, M. T., Howell, E. F., Ballenger, J. C.: Can panic disorder present as irritable bowel syndrome? J Clin Psychiatry 1986, 47: 470–473.
[5] Walker, E. A., Katon, W. J., Jemelka, R. P., Roy-Byrne, P. P.: Comorbidity of gastrointestinal complaints, depression, and anxiety in the epidemiologic catchment area (ECA) Study. Am J Med 1992, 92: 26S–30S.
[6] Lydiard, R. B., Greenwald, S., Weissman, M. M., Johnnson, J.; Drossman, D. A., Ballenger, J. C.: Panic disorder and gastrointestinal symptoms: Findings from the NIMH Epidemiologic Catchment Area project. Am J Psychiatry 1994, 151: 64–70.
[7] Whitehead, W. E., Bosmajian, L., Zonderman, A. B., Costa, P. T., Schuster, M. M.: Symptoms of psychologic distress associated with irritable bowel syndrome: comparison of community and medical clinic samples. Gastroenterology 1988, 95: 709–714.
[8] Blanchard, E. B., Scharff, L., Schwarz, S. P., Suls, J. M., Barlow, D. H.: The role of anxiety and depression in the irritable bowel syndrome. Behav Res Ther 1990, 28: 401–405.
[9] Latimer, P. R.: Irritable bowel syndrome: a behavioural model. Behav Res Ther 1981, 19: 475–483.
[10] Walker, E. A., Roy-Byrne, P. P., Katon, W.: Irritable bowel syndrome and psychiatric illness. Am J Psychiatry 1990, 147: 565–572.
[11] Sandler, R. S., Drossman, D. A., Nathan, H. P., McKee, D. C.: Symptom complaints and health care seeking behavior in subjects with bowel dysfunction. Gastroenterology 1984, 87: 314–318.
[12] Longstreth, G. F., Wolde-Tsadik, G.: Irritable bowel-type symptoms in HMO examinees. Dig Dis Sci 1993, 38: 1581–1589.
[13] Veale, D., Kavanagh, G., Fielding, J. F., Fitzgerald, O.: Primary fibromyalgia and the irritable bowel syndrome: different expressions of a common pathogenetic process. Br J Rheumatol 1991, 30: 220–222.
[14] Triadafilopoulos, G., Simms, R. W., Goldenberg, D. L.: Bowel dysfunction in fibromyalgia syndrome. Dig Dis Sci 1991, 36: 59–64.
[15] Crowell, M. D., Dubin, N. H., Robinson, J. C., Cheskin, L. J., Schuster, M. M., Heller, B. R., Whitehead, W. E.: Functional bowel disorders in women with dysmenorrhea. Am J Gastroenterol 1994, 89: 1973–1977.
[16] Prior, A., Whorwell, P. J.: Gynaecological consultation in patients with the irritable bowel syndrome. Gut 1989, 30: 996–998.
[17] Whorwell, P. J., Lupton, E. W., Erduran, D., Wilson, K.: Bladder smooth muscle dysfunction in patients with irritable bowel syndrome. Gut 1986, 27: 1014–1017.
[18] Whorwell, P. J., McCallum, M., Creed, F. H., Roberts, C. T.: Non-colonic features of irritable bowel syndrome. Gut 1986, 27: 37–40.
[19] Drossman, D. A., Li, L., Andruzzi, e., Temple, R., Talley, N. J., Thompson, W. G., Whitehead, W. E., Janssens, J., Funch-Jensen, P., Corazziari, E., Richter, E., Koch, G. G.: US householder survey of functional gastrointestinal disorders. Prevalence, sociodemography and health impact. Dig Dis Sci 1993, 38: 1569–1580.
[20] Whitehead, W. E., Cheskin, L. J., Heller, B. R., Robinson, J. C., Crowell, M. D., Benjamin, C., Schuster, M. M., Evidence for exacerbation of irritable bowel syndrome during menses. Gastroenterology 1990, 98: 1485–1489.
[21] Longstreth, G. F., Preskill, D. B., Youkles, L.: Irritable bowel syndrome in women having diagnostic laparoscopy or hysterectomy. Relation to gynecoilogic features and outcome. Dig Dis Sci 1990, 35: 1285–1290.

[22] Mechanic, D.: Adolescent health and illness behavior: review of the literature and a new hypothesis for the study of stress. J Hum Stress 1983, 9: 4–13.
[23] Whitehead, W. E., Holtkotter, B., Enck, P., Hoelzl, R., Holmes, K. D., Anthony, J., Shabsin, H. S., Schuster, M. M.: Tolerance for rectosigmoid distension in irritable bowel syndrome. Gastroenterology 1990, 98: 1187–1192.
[24] Kellow, J. E., Langeluddecke, P. M., Eckersley, G. M., Jones, M. P., Tennant, C. C.: Effects of acute psychologic stress on small-intestinal motility in health and the irritable bowel syndrome. Scand J Gastroenterol 1992, 27: 53–58.
[25] Kellow, J. E., Phillips, S. F.: Altered small bowel motility in irritable bowel syndrome is correlated with symptoms. Gastroenterology 1987, 92: 1885–1893.
[26] Mertz, H., Naliboff, B., Munakata, J., Niazi, N., Mayer, E. A.: Altered rectal perception is a biological marker of patients with irritable bowel syndrome. Gastroenterology 1995, 109: 40–52.
[27] Almy, T. P.: Experimental studies on the irritable colon. Am J Medicine 1951, 9: 60–67.
[28] Kellner, R., Hernandez, J., Pathak, D.: Hypochondriacal, fears and beliefs, anxiety, and somatization. Br J Psychiatry 1992, 160: 525–532.
[29] Drossman, D. A., McKee, D. C., Sandler, R. S., Mitchell, C. M., Cramer, E. M., Lowman, B. C., Berger, A. L.: Psychological factors in the irritable bowel syndrome. A multivariate study of patients and nonpatients with irritable bowel syndrome. Gastroenterology 1988, 95: 701–708.
[30] Whitehead, W. E., Crowell, M. D., Bosmajian, L., Zonderman, A., Costa, P. T. Jr., Robinson, I. C., Heller, B. R., Schuster, M. M.: Existence of irritable bowel syndrome supported by factor analysis of symptoms in two community samples. Gastroenterology 1990, 98: 336–340.
[31] Taub, E., Cuevas, J. L., Cook, E. W. III, Crowell, M., Whitehead, W. E.: Irritable bowel syndrome defined by factor analysis: gender and race comparisons. Dig Dis Sci 1995, 40: 2647–2655.
[32] Trimble, K. C., Farouk, R., Pryde, A., Douglas, S., Heading, R. C.: Heightened visceral sensation in functional gastrointestinal disease is not site-specific. Evidence for a generalized disorder of gut sensitivity. Dig Dis Sci 1995, 40: 1607–1613.
[33] Whitehead, W. E.: Functional bowel disorders: Are they independent diagnoses? In: Corazziari, E. (ed.), Neurogastroenterology. W. de Gruyter, Berlin 1996.
[34] Agreus, L., Svardsudd, K., Nyren, O., Tibblin, G.: Irritable bowel syndrome and dyspepsia in the general population: Overlap and lack of stability over time. Gastroenterology 1994, 109: 671–680.
[35] Palsson, O., Taub, E., Cook, E. C. III, Burnett, C. K., McCommons, J. J., Whitehead, W. E.: Validation of the Rome criteria for functional gastrointestinal disorders by factor analysis. Am J Gastroenterol 1996, 91: A 2000.
[36] Drossman, D. A., Richter, J. E., Talley, N. J., Thompson, W. G., Corazziari, E., Whitehead, W. E.: The functional gastrointestinal disorders: Diagnosis, pathophysiology, and treatment. Boston, Little, Brown & Co, 1994.
[37] Talley, N. J., Zinsmeister, A. R., Schleck, C. D., Melton, L. J. III: Dyspepsia and dyspepsia subgroups: a population-based study. Gastroenterology 1992, 102: 1259–1268.
[38] Smith, R. C., Greenbaum, D. S., Vancouver, J. B., Henry, R. C., Reinhart, M. A., Greenbaum, R. B., Dean, I. A., Mayle, J. E.: Psychosocial factors are associated with health care seeking rather than diagnosis in irritable bowel syndrome. Gastroenterology 1990, 98: 293–301.
[39] Drossman, D. A., McKee, D. C., Sandler, R. S., Mitchell, C. M., Cramer, E. M., Lowman et al.: Psychological factors in the irritable bowel syndrome. A multivariate study of patients and nonpatients with irritable bowel syndrome. Gastroenterology 1988, 95: 701–708.

[40] Whitehead, W. E., Crowell, M. D., Robinson, J. C., Heller, B. R., Schuster, M. M.: Effects of stressful life events on bowel symptoms: subjects with irritable bowel syndrome compared with subjects without bowel dysfunction. Gut 1992, 33: 825–830.
[41] Ford, M. J., Miller, P. M., Eastwood, J., Eastwood, M. A.: Life events, psychiatric illness and the irritable bowel syndrome. Gut 1987, 28: 160–165.
[42] Hislop, I. G.: Psychological significance of the irritable colon syndrome. Gut 1971, 12: 452–457.
[43] Whitehead, W. E., Burnett, C. K., Cook, E. W. III, Taub, E.: Impact of irritable bowel syndrome on quality of life. Dig Dis Sci. in press.
[44] Hill, O. W., Blendis, L.: Physical and psychological evaluation of 'non-organis' abdominal pain. Gut 1967, 8: 221–229.
[45] Hislop, I. G.: Childhood deprivation: An antecedent of the irritable bowel syndrome. Gut 1971, 12: 452–457.
[46] Lowman, B. C., Drossman, D. A., Cramer, E. M., McKee, D. C.: Recollection of childhood events in adults with irritable bowel syndrome. J Clin Gastroenterol 1987, 9: 324–330.
[47] Drossman, D. A., Leserman, J., Nachman, G., Li, Z., Gluck, H., Toomey, T. C., Mitchell, M.: Sexual and physical abuse in women with functional or organic gastrointestinal disorders. Ann Int Med 1990, 113: 828–833.
[48] Talley, N. J., Fett, S. L., Zinsmeister, A. R., Melton, L. J. III: Gastrointestinal tract symptoms and self-reported abuse: A population-based study. Gastroenterology 1994, 107: 1040–1049.
[49] Drossman, D. A., Talley, N. J., Leserman, J., Olden, K. W., Barreiro, M. A.: Sexual and physical abuse and gastrointestinal illness: Review and recommendations. Ann Intern Med 1995, 123: 782–794.
[50] Whitehead, W. E., Winget, C., Fedoravicius, A. S. et al.: Learned illness behavior in patients with irritable bowel syndrome and peptic ulcer. Dig Dis Sci 1982, 27: 202–208.
[51] Whitehead, W. E., Busch, C. M., Heller, B. R., Costa, P. T. Jr.: Social leraning influences on menstrual symptoms and illness behavior. Health Psychol 1986, 5: 13–23.
[52] Whitehead, W. E., Crowell, M. D., Heller, B. R., Robinson, J. C., Schuster, M. M., Horn, S.: Modeling and reinforcement of the sick role during childhood predicts adult illness behavior. Psychosomatic Medicine 1994, 56: 541–550.

Abdominal pain in gastrointestinal disorders – differences between IBS and other gastrointestinal disorders

H. Bosseckert

Epidemiological studies prove that irritable bowel syndrome (IBS) represents the most frequent somatoform disorder. In addition, functional disorders of IBS is the most common. Nevertheless, we have to keep in mind that – like in esophageal reflux disease – a significant proportion of those persons not seek medical care, i. e., there exists an iceberg phenomenon in IBS, too. Consultation behavior was influenced by age, use of laxatives and presence of associated symptoms [1–3].

The absence of positive criteria for the diagnosis of IBS allows for diagnosis only by means of exclusion criteria. But the great number of patients who suffer from complaints of IBS – about 30% of all referrals to a clinic of gastroenterology – demands a preliminary decision as to whether an extensive program for diagnosis will be necessary or not.

Perhaps proctometrography is one step in the direction of developing positive criteria for diagnosis of IBS [4] (tab. 1). Intracolic injection of glycerol which triggers viscerovisceral reflexes, resulting in abdominal pain may be yet another one [5].

Table 1 Fluidinfusion proctometrography and visceral hypersensitivity in IBS

	Patients	Control subj.
Threshold vol.	129 ± 8	229 ± 24
Constant sensation vol.	159 ± 12	286 ± 21
Max. tolerance vol.	290 ± 13	509 ± 19

Varma, J. S., Smith, A. N. [4]

The principal symptoms of IBS are recurrent or continuous abdominal pains in relation to disturbed defecation which can not be explained by structural or biochemical deviations. Therefore, IBS is a clinical syndrome of uncertain etiology and has to be classified as a functional bowel disease. According to the so-called Rome criteria, IBS belongs to the subcategories of functional bowel disorders group C 1.

The international classification scheme (WHO) ICD-10 defines the IBS as a somatoform autonome functional disorder of the lower gastrointestinal tract.

Symptomatology

Abdominal pain or discomfort vary in intensity, nature and location. Goldsmith and Levin [6] for instance observed in their study that a bad quality in sleeping was related with a higher symptom score of complaints in IBS patients although there is noctural well-being and the patient does not feel the symptoms when he sleeps.

The pain may worsen after getting up in the morning or half an hour or so after eating. These events have been correlated with specific bursts of motility in the small intestine and arrival of luminal contents in the caecum (Evans [7]). On the other hand, some IBS patients experience rather constant pain. These patients often belong to the group of patients who respond poorly to most treatments [8].

The pain can be exacerbated by a number of factors with stress at the fore most. In a group of subjects not seeking health care but who reported disorders of bowel motility, the group of females more often exhibited an influence of stress on their bowel function [2]. It has been shown (Kollmannsperger et al. [9]) that mental stress leads to an increased rectal tone and a greater increase for the motility index in the rectum as well as the anal high pressure zone in IBS patients to the controls.

Since stress events are relatively temporary, the symptoms of IBS may be worsened only at certain times.

Gastrointestinal infections and drugs are additional factors which trigger the painful symptoms of IBS. The same holds true for cleansing of the large bowel and even sigmoido- or colonoscopy. Interestingly, in some patients who have normal perception thresholds during balloon distension discomfort or pain can be evoked by sigmoidoscopy or pulling through an inflated balloon through the sigmoid colon [10].

The pain in IBS can occur anywhere in the abdominal region and may be the reason for false diagnosis (fig. 1). The considerable overlap between organic intestinal disorders and IBS is of important concern.

Differential diagnosis to other gastrointestinal disorders

If the pain is localized in the *lower left quadrant* diverticulitis, ulcerative colitis, Crohn's disease, ischemic colitis, sigmoid cancer, urogenital disease, endometriosis have to be excluded.

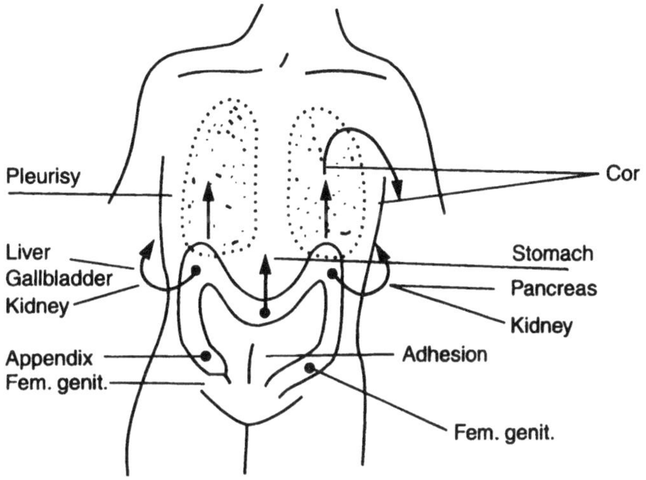

Abb. 1 Radiation of pains due to IBS

Pain in the *lower right quadrant* demands a differential diagnosis for appendicitis, Crohn's disease, yersiniosis, ureterolithiasis or urogenital disease.

Gall stone disease or cholecystitis, kidney disease, duodenal ulcers and pleurisy have to be excluded if the pain is localized in the *right upper side* of abdomen.

Symptoms in the left upper side of abdomen in IBS patients can simulate pancreatitis, ulcerative colitis, Crohn's disease, ischemic colitis or splenitis.

In our experiences, however, the pain is often registered in the epigastric region and can be relieved by palpation of the transverse colon. That is one point which explains the great overlap with functional dyspepsia.

In a very recent study Agreus et al. [11] showed that 87% of patients with core symptoms fulfilling the symptom criteria for IBS also had symptoms fulfilling the criteria for functional dyspepsia. In addition, functional dyspepsia as well as IBS are both characterized by altered small bowel mechanosensitive pathways [12]. Kellow et al. [13] found a significantly greater rate of occurrence of abdominal sensation in patients with IBS than in controls. These episodes occurred during duodenal phase 3 activity and these activity fronts were of significantly higher amplitude. The results of the study lead to the conclusion that the perception of intestinal contractions is lower in a number of patients with IBS.

Similar results have been demonstrated by Accarino et al. [14], but they found even a reduced somatic sensitivity in patients with IBS.

But, in addition to functional dyspepsia, we have to realize that ischemias of the small and large bowel, cancer of the pancreas, of transverse colon or of the

Table 2 Principal signs and symptoms used in the diagnosis of IBS and those commonly seen in patients with organic gastrointestinal disorders[a]

Symptom	IBS	Ulceratice Colitis	Crohn's disease	Diverticulitis	Colorectal cancer
Abdominal pain or discomfort	+	+	+	+	+
Altered stool frequency (e. g. diarrhea, constipation)	+	+	+	+	+
Altered stool form (lumpy/ hard, loose/watery)	+	+	+	+	+
Altered stool passage (straining, urgency, feeling of incomplete evacuation)	+	+			+
Passage of mucus	+				
Bloating, feeling of abdominal distension	+	+			+
Other		Passage of blood Passage of pus Fever Weight loss	Fatigue Fever Weight loss	Fever Muscle spasm, Guarding Tenderness	Passage of blood Nausea/ vomiting Fatigue Congestive heart failure

[a] Signs and symptoms depend on the severity, extent and/or location of disease
(after Cohnen et al. [26], Glickman [27], La Mont and Isselbacher [28], Mayer [10], Thompson et al. [25, 29]

stomach (especially scirrhus cancer, which is sometimes difficult to diagnose) may mimic IBS.

The most principal signs and symptoms used in the diagnosis of IBS and those seen in patients with organic large bowel disease are very similar (tab. 2). A number of other symptoms are helpful in differentiation: weight loss, fever, passage of blood and pus, guarding tenderness. The so-called painful diverticular disease, i. e., the development of colic-like abdominal pain which often is relieved by defecation or by passage of flatus is the expression of IBS *and* diverticular disease where diverticular disease may be the consequence of IBS.

There is also an overlap of functional constipation, outlet delay and IBS (tab. 3). In an age- and gender stratified random sample of residents of Olmstedt county with the main symptom of constipation Talley et al. [15] observed an overlap of the three syndromes in 35% of subjects. By a step-wise logistic regression analysis they found the following symptoms (tab. 4) associated with functional constipation:

painful defecation, feeling of anal blockage, prolonged defecation, manual disimpaction, fecal incontinence, and postprandial abdominal bloating ($p < 0.05$).

Table 3 Principal symptoms used in the diagnosis of IBS and other functional gastrointestinal disorders

Symptom	IBS	Functional constipation	Functional diarrhoea	Functional dyspepsia
Abdominal pain or discomfort	+			+
Altered stool frequency (e. g. diarrhoea, constipation)	+	+	+	
Altered stool form (lumpy/hard, loose/ watery)	+	+	+	
Altered stool passage (straining, urgency, feeling of incomplete evacuations	+	+	+	
Passage of mucous	+			
Bloating, feeling of abdominal distension	+			
Other				Reflux Heartburn Pain behind the breastbone Belching Nausea/vomiting Early satiety

(after Thompson et al. [25, 30], Colin-Jones et al. [31])

Table 4 Gastrointestinal symptoms in functional constipation

- painful defecation
- feeling of anal blockage
- prolonged defecation
- manual disimpaction
- fecal incontinence
- postprandial abdominal bloating

Talley et al. [15]

In outlet delay, the only symptom which was identified multivariantly was straining. Narcotic bowel syndrome [16], pseudo-obstruction, amyloidosis, systemic scleroderma, carcinoid syndrome and other systemic diseases have to be considered in differential diagnosis to IBS.

In addition to the symptoms mentioned or signs in relation to IBS, there is an association with a number of functional disorders or vegetative signs like globus sensation, fatigue, sleeping disturbancies, tendency for sweating, non-cardiac chest pain, biliary diskinesia, proctalgia fugax, fibromyalgia. Taking these complaints into consideration, an experienced clinician has further hints for diagnosis of functional disease.

In order to support the efforts to make a positive diagnosis of IBS, the *Manning* criteria were developed in 1978. The following signs allow differentation from organic diseases:

- Looser stools with onset of pain ($p < 0.001$),
- More frequent stools with onset of pain ($p < 0.01$),
- Abdominal pain or discomfort relieved with defecation ($p < 0.01$),
- Abdominal distention ($p < 0.01$),
- Passage of mucous,
- Sensation of incomplete evacuation,
- Feeling of abdominal distention.

In 1990, Whitehead et al. [18] investigated the question of whether IBS exists as a distinct syndrome by collecting reports from women who were not characterized through their attendance at medical clinics. They identified four signs, from which three correspond to the first three of Manning and the fourth sign was gastrointestinal reactions to eating. A gender difference of diagnosis of IBS using the Manning criteria was reported by Smith et al. [19]. The results show that the Manning criteria were not of diagnostic help in men.

Another study by Kruis et al. [20] used a detailed history, physical examination and basic laboratory tests for the positive diagnosis of IBS and exclusion of underlying organic diseases. The score consists of two parts, from which the first part has to be filled out by the patient (tab. 5) and the second part (abnormal clinical findings and/or a pathognomonic history for any diagnosis other than IBS by the physician. Laboratory parameters are ESR, leucocytosis, hemoglobin and history of blood in stool. Though the method seems to allow a good differentiation between organic disease and IBS, it did not gain wide acceptance because it is not easyly applicable in clinical practice.

Table 5 Kruis' index for diagnosis of IBS [20]

Questions to be answered by the patient	
1. Did you come because of abdominal pain? Do you suffer from flatulence? Do you suffer from irregularities of bowel movement?	34
2. Have you suffered from your complaints for more than two years?	16
3. How can your abdominal pain be described: burning, cutting, very strong, terrible, feeling of pressure, dull, borinng, not so bad?	23
4. Have you noticed alternating constipation and diarrhea?	14

Table 6 Diagnostic criteria for IBS: Rome criteria [32]

Continuous or recurrent symptoms for at least three months of:

1. abdominal pain or discomfort, relieved with defecation, or associated with a change in frequency or consistency of stool;

and

2. an irregular (varying) pattern of defecation at least 25% of the time (three or more of):
   altered stool frequency;
   altered stool form (hard or loose/watery stool);
   altered stool passage (straining or urgency, feeling of incomplete evacuation);
   passage of mucous;
   bloating or feeling of abdominal distension

Based on the Manning criteria, the so-called Rome criteria were accepted during a consensus conference in Rome 1988 (tab. 6) [32]. They consist of the following symptoms: Abdominal pain or discomfort relieved with defecation or associated with a change in frequency or consistency of stools, an irregular pattern of defecation at least 25% of time consisting of three (changed in a later consensus into "two") [32] or more of the following: altered stool frequency, altered stool form, altered stool passage and bloating or feeling of abdominal distention.

A more accurate diagnosis of IBS might be possible if "non-colonic" symptomatology is taken in consideration. Maxton et al. [21] reported that the following features (tab. 7) are of particular value in assessing the relative risk of IBS: Lethargy, incomplete evacuation, age less than 40 years, backache, early satiety, frequency of micturation. If a patient who may have IBS also showed non-colonic symptoms, i. e., lethargy, incomplete evacuation and early satiety, the relative risk factors can be multiplied together ($6.7 \times 5.2 \times 1.8 = 67.7$) and making IBS much more likely than organic disease. It is remarkable that the discriminant value and relative risk of all the non-colonic symptoms, apart from

Table 7 Relative risk of specific clinical features for irritable bowel syndrome vs organic gastrointestinal disease [21]

Feature	Relative risk	95% confidence interval
1. Lethargy	6.7	3.4 to 13.3
2. Incomplete evacuation	5.2	2.9 to 9.2
3. Age less than 40 years	2.1	1.2 to 3.8
4. Backache	2.0	1.1 to 3.8
5. Early satiety	1.8	1.1 to 3.2
6. Frequency of micturition	1.8	1.0 to 3.1

those relating to frequency of micturation, seemed to be independent of gender. Four of the non-colonic symptoms are vegetative signs which have been mentioned above.

In a recent study by Müller-Lissner's working group [22] it was shown that by use of a functional diagnostic work-up (functional proctoscopy, defecography, anorectal manometry, colonic transit of radiopague markers and lactose tolerance test) a diagnosis could be made in 52% of the patients suffering from IBS. They found in another 10% of patients their sample organic diseases by means of a conventional diagnostic work-up. The evaluation of symptoms with a standardized questionnaire revealed "constipation" and "straining" as very specific for IBS (93% and 100%), but the sensitivity of the two symptoms reached only 64% and 53% respectively (tab. 8)[22]. Surprinsingly, the Manning criteria in the sample examined were not discriminatory. Nevertheless, it is worth noting that the results of the study may have been affected by selection bias due to referral of many constipated patients to the investigators. The study shows that the use of functional tests can lead to a specific diagnosis in more than half of the patients who primarily were diagnosed as IBS patients. But in order to make these specific diagnoses it will be neccessary for spreading these functional tests.

Table 8 Symptoms which reached significance and their discriminatory value for IBS [22]

	Organic disease	IBS	p
Diarrhea	86% (79%)	30% (22%)	0.001
Constipation	7% (0%)	64% (60%)	0.001
Straining	0% (0%)	53% (3%)	0.002
Hard stools	7% (0%)	43% (0%)	0.01
Metorism	21% (7%)	59% (3%)	0.01
Abdominal pain	100% (14%)	100% (4%)	

However, there are other studies to support the diagnosis of IBS by endoscopic signs. Matek et al. [23] found the following features for this: The lumen of the large bowel must be temporarily closed, the functional stenosis has to be sustained at least 15 seconds and during total colonoscopy at least five such spasms should be observed. Perhaps one can added to these signs the symptom of pain produced by movements of the endoscope and/or a special sensitivity for air insufflation. Until now there is no evident agreement for the recommendation of colonoscopy in the diagnosis of IBS. The point of view varies as to whether a practioner or a clinician has to make the decision. If a patient is referred to the clinic a colonoscopy should be performed because of the ultimate responsibility. As a common recommendation one can say, when a patient is older than fifty years, the diagnosis of IBS without performing a total colonoscopy should not be made.

IBS is associated with a good prognosis when diagnosed according to current criteria. The therapeutic effectiveness of a positive physician-patient interaction is revealed through a reduction in use of ambulatory health services [24].

Table 9 Steps in diagnosis of IBS

- Ask for "vegetative" signs!

↓

- Check the Rome criteria

↓

- Are there symptoms for organic disease?

↓

- How is the lactose-, sorbitol- or fructose intolerance

↓

- Which drugs does the patient use?

↓

- Decide about a colonoscopic examination!

In summary, recurrent or continuous pain in relation to disturbed defecation in patients who show some vegatative signs like lethargy, globus sensation, tendency for sweating, backache, early satiety, non-cardiac chest pain, sleeping disturbancies and others should be asked if typical symptoms for IBS have been present for more than three months (tab. 9). Then check for the presence of the Rome criteria and exclude symptoms which give hints of organic disease. In addition, it is advisable to ask for lactose-, sorbitol- oder fructose intolerance as well as medications which could evoke abdominal disturbancies. If there is some doubt concerning the diagnosis of IBS or if a patient with more than 50 years of age suffers from symptoms of IBS for the first time or reveals carcinophobia a colonoscopy should be performed, because it is more certain and often an important part of the therapeutic armament.

References

[1] Thompson, W. G., Heaton, K. W.: Functional bowel disorders in apparently healthy people. Gastroenterology 1980, 79: 283–288.

[2] Drossman, D. A., Sandler, R. S., McKee, Daphne C., Lovitz, A. J.: Bowel patterns among subjects not seeking health care. Gastroenterology 1982, 83: 529–534.

[3] Jones, R., Lydeard, S.: Irritable bowel syndrome in the general population. Br Med J 1992, 304: 87–90.

[4] Varma, J. S., Smith, A. N.: Reproducibility of the proctometrogram. Gut 1986, 27: 288–292.

[5] Louvel, D., Delvaux, M., Staumont, G., Camman, F., Fioramonti, J., Bueno, L., Frexinos, J.: Intracolonic Injection of Glycerol: A model for abdominal pain in irritable bowel syndrome? Gastroenterology 1996, 110: 351–361.

[6] Goldsmith, G., Levin, S. J.: Effect of sleep quality on symptoms of irritable bowel syndrome. Dig Dis Sci 1993, 10: 1809–1814.

[7] Evans, P. R., ennett, E. J., Bak, Y.-T., Tennant, C. C., Kellow, J. E.: Jejunal sensorimotor dysfunction in irritable bowel syndrome: Clinical and psychosocial features. Gastroenterology 1996, 110: 393–404.

[8] Guthrie, Elspeth, Creed, F., Dawson, D., Tomenson, B.: A controlled trial of psychological treatment for the irritable bowel syndrome. Gastroenterology 1991, 100: 450–457.

[9] Kollmannsperger, P., Musiai, F., Mueller, J., Crowell, M. D.: Mental stress affects rectal tone, anorectal motility and autonomic function in patients with the irritable bowel syndrome. Gastroenterology 1994, 105: 1020 Abstr.)

[10] Mayer, E. A.: Gut Feelings: What turns them on? Gastroenterology 1995, 108: 927–940.

[11] Agreus, L., Svärdsudd, K., Nyren, O., Tibblin, G.: Irritable bowel syndrome and dyspepsia in the generalpopulation: overlap and lack of stability over time. Gastroenterology 1995, 109: 671–680.

[12] Holtmann, G., Goebell, H., Talley., N. J.: Functional dyspepsia and irritable bowel syndrome: clinical and experimentale edivence for a common pathophysiologic basis. Gut 1995, 36: A 37.

[13] Kellow, J. E., Eckersley, G. M., Jones, M. P.: Enhanced perception of physiological intestinal motility in the irritable bowel syndrome. Gastroenterology 1991, 10: 1621–1627.

[14] Accarino, A., Azpiroz, F., Malagelada, J.-R.: Selective dysfunction of mechanosensitive intestinal afferents in irritable bowel syndrome. Gastroenterology 1995, 108: 636–643.

[15] Talley, N. J., Weaver, A. L., Zinsmeister, A. R., Melton, L.-J.: Functional constipation and outlet delay: A population-based study. Gastroenterology 1993, 105: 781–790.

[16] Sandgren, J. E., McPhee, M. S., Greenberger, N. J.: Narcotic bowel syndrome treated with clonidine. Ann Intern Med 1984, 10: 331–334.

[17] Manning, A. P., Thompson, W. G., Heaton, K. W., Morris, A. F.: Towards positive diagnosis of the irritable bowel. Br Med J 1978, II, 653–654.

[18] Whitehead, W. E., Crowell, M. D., Bosjajian, L., Zondermann, A., Costa, P. T. Jr., Benjamin, C., Robinson, J. C., Heller, B. R., Schuster, M. M.: Existence of irritable bowel syndrome supported by factor analysis of symptoms in two community samples. Gastroenterology 1990, 98: 336–340.

[19] Smith, R. C., Greenbaum, D. S., Vancouver, J. B., Henry, R. C., Reinhart, M. A., Greenbaum, R. B., Dean, H. A., Mayle, J. E.: Gender differences in Manning criteria in the irritable bowel syndrome. Gastroenterology 1991, 100: 591–595.

[20] Kruis, W., Thieme, Ch., Weinzierl, M., Schüssler, P., Holl, J., Paulus, W.: A diagnostic score for the irritable bowel syndrome. Gastroenterology 1984, 87: 11–17.

[21] Maxton, D. G., Morris, J., Whorwell, P. J.: More accurate diagnosis of irritable bowel syndrome by the use of "non-colonic" symptomatology. Gut 1991, 32: 784–786.

[22] Klauser, A. G., Voderholzer, W. A., Schindlbeck, N. E., Müller-Sissner, S. A.: Functional diagnostic work-up in patients with irritable bowel syndrome. Z Gastroenterol 1996, 34: 273–278.

[23] Matek, W., Frühmorgen, P., Demling, L.: Endoskop.-diagn. Möglichkeiten beim Colon irritable. Dtsch Med Wschr 1982, 107: 375–377.

[24] Owens, D. M., Nelson, D. K., Talley, N. J.: The irritable bowel syndrome: Long-term prognosis and the physician-patient interaction. Ann. Intern Med. 1995, 122: 107–112.

[25] Thompson, W. G., Dotevall, G., Drossman, D.A. et al.: Irritable bowel syndrome: Guidelines for the diagnosis. Gastroenterol Int 1989, 2: 92–95.

[26] Cohen, A. M., Minsky, B. D., Schilsky, R. L.: Colon cancer. In: DeVita, V. T., Jr., Hellman, S., Rosenberg, S. A. (eds.), Cancer: Principles and practise of oncology. 4th edition, Philadelphia, Lippincott, 1993, 929–977.

[27] Glickman, R. M.: Inflammatory bowel disease: Ulcerative colitis and Crohn's disease. In: Wilson, J. D., Braunwald, E., Isselbacher, K. J. et al. (eds.), Harrison's principles of interal medicine. 12th edition, New York, McGraw-Hill, 1991: 1268–1281.

[28] LaMont, J. T., Isselbacher, K. J.: Diseases of the small and large intestine. In: Wilson, J. D., Braunwald, E., Isselbacher, K. J. et al. (eds.), Harrison's principles of interal medicine. 12th edition, New York, McGraw-Hill, 1991: 1268–1281.

[29] Thompson W. G., Creed, F., Drossman, D. A. et al.: Functional bowel disease and functional abdominal pain. Gastroenterol Int 1992, 5: 75–91.

[30] Colin-Jones, D., Bloom, B., Bodemar, G., Crean, G., Freston, J., Gugler, R., Malagelada, J., Nyrén, O., Petersen, H., Piper, D.: Management of dyspepsia: Report of a working party. Lancet 1988, 1: 576–579.

[31] Drossman, D. A., Thompson W. G., Talley, N. J., Funch-Jensen, P., Janssens, J., Whitehead, W. E.: Identification of sub-groups of functional gastrointestinal disorders. Gastroenterol Int 1990, 3: 159–172.

Visceral sensitivity: What are the perspectives for the clinician?

M. Delvaux

Functional digestive disorders include a number of syndromes which have recently been characterized by a visceral hypersensitivity underlying painful perception of abdominal sensations. Visceral hypersensitivity is detected mainly by distension studies of the gut. The recognition of visceral hypersensitivity as one of the critical features underlying the pathophysiology of functional digestive disorders has been the main advance over the last decade in the understanding of these conditions and has shed light on the role of visceral afferents from the gut. This new concept has led to a number of studies, dealing with either basic or clinical science, the results of which are intended to bring new insights in the diagnosis and treatment of these functional bowel disorders.

A diffuse and multimodal disorder

Abdominal hypersensitivity can be defined as the exaggerated perception of various stimuli in different segments of the digestive tract. Among them, luminal distension of hollow organs has been the most studied. Since 1975, Lasser and coll. have shown that patients with irritable bowel syndrome (IBS) tolerated lower volumes of gas infused in the ileum than controls [1]. Balloon distension [2] and recently barostat studies [3], which allow more precise and reproducible results from distension protocols, have shown that gut hypersensitivity is more diffuse than limited to the digestive segment classically thought to be responsible for the disorder, whatever the symptoms claimed by the patients [4]. Visceral hypersensitivity is also common to any kind of functional digestive disorder and is found in IBS patients als well as in functional diarrhea, non-ulcer dyspepsia [5] and non-cardiac chest pain patients [6].

Other stimuli than luminal distension can also generate abnormal painful sensations in patients with functional digestive disorders, like lipid infusion into the duodenum [7] or infusion of hyperosmotic food in the oesophagus in patients with non-cardiac chest pain [8]. Moreover, some studies have shown that patients with functional bowel disorders perceived abdominal events usually not perceived by controls, such as physiological contractions of the jejunum [9] or oesophageal endoscopic biopsies [10].

How can visceral hypersensitivity be integrated in clinical practice?

Pathophysiology of functional bowel disorders is obviously multifactorial at the moment. Many factors are indeed associated in determining the onset of symptoms in a given patient. Beside visceral hypersensitivity, motility disorders play a role, although they are not constantly observed and unspecific. They are found in many patients at the gastric, intestinal and recto-colonic levels. Psychosocial factors like depression, anxiety, stress and personal background of the patient – physical and sexual abuse – are also of importance.

Many questions remain unsolved. The primary anomaly underlying visceral hypersensitivity is not clearly known. Some studies have shed light on the role of mechanical receptors of the abdominal wall [11] while others emphasized on the afferent pathways [12]. Recent studies using the PET scanner, i. e., computerized cerebral tomography by positron emission, have shown abnormalities of brain perception of abdominal sensations in IBS patients [13] and the abnormal activation of some thalamic areas in these patients during rectal distension tests [14]. From these results, it becomes clear that processing of painful sensations originating from the gut or perception of sensations as painful ones by the brain are complex matters, where each level of the nerve pathways may play a role. Moreover, at each level, connections link afferent and efferent pathways and allow reflexes which may themselves trigger an hypersensitive reaction (see below).

The frequent observation of visceral hypersensitivity in patients with functional bowel disorders led to it being considered a basic mechanism underlying the

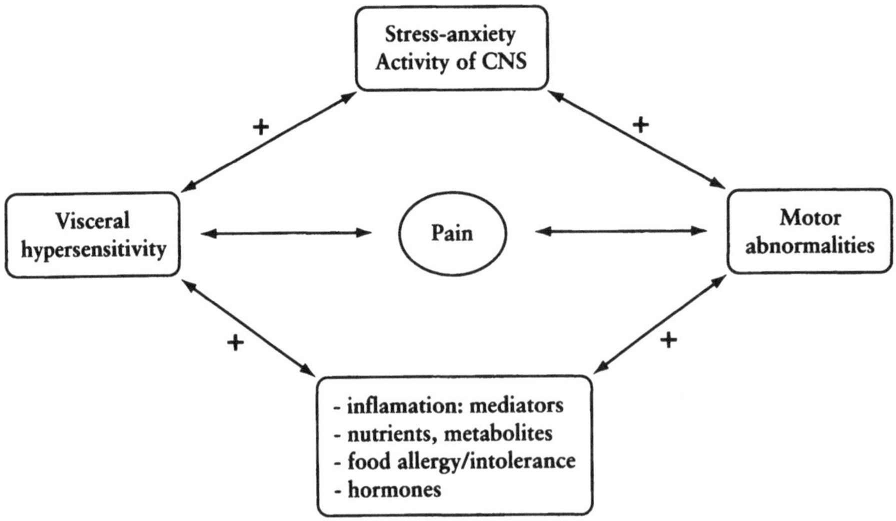

Fig. 1 Relationship between functional bowel disorders and visceral hypersensitivity

pathophysiology of these disorders (fig. 1). However, the relationship between functional bowel disorders and visceral hypersensitivity is not unequivocal. The question whether visceral hypersensitivity is cause or consequence of functional bowel disorders is unanswered. Indeed, about one third of IBS patients, perfectly fulfilling the Rome criteria [15] are not hypersensitive to rectal distension [12, 16]. Among IBS patients, those with functional diarrhea seem to be more frequently hypersensitive than the constipated ones [17] and an acute diarrhea can by itself induce rectal hypersensitivity to distension in healthy volunteers [18]. Visceral hypersensitivity appears thus to be influenced by a number of factors (tab. 1). Most interesting is the observation by Mertz et al. who studied a small number of IBS patients [19] several times. They observed that visceral hypersensitivity was directly linked to the intensity of IBS-related symptoms, the more symptomatic patients being the more sensitive. In view of these results, one could consider visceral hypersensitivity as a marker of the intensity of symptoms, the primary disorder underlying both the symptoms and the hypersensitivity remaining unknown.

Table 1 Factors influencing perception thresholds of luminal distension.

Age
Sex, phase of the menstrual cycle in women?
Tone of the organ
Stress, anxiety
Protocol of distension
Intensity of IBS-related symptoms

The present knowledge does not allow only one mechanism for the onset of visceral hypersensitivity in a single patient to be proposed. Psycho-social factors are of importance. Rectal hypersensitivity is more frequently observed in patients threatened with sexual abuse [20]. Stress and anxiety may also influence perception of rectal and colonic sensations [21]. Among the factors that can trigger a visceral hypersensitivity, researchers have recently focused attention on mucosal inflammation. Several studies have demonstrated the existence of abnormalities of inflammatory mediators or of immune cells in patients with functional bowel disorders (22).

During inflammation, a number of substances are released in the gut wall, including K^+ ions and neuromediators like bradykinin, substance P, serotonin, histamine, prostaglandins. These mediators interact in a complex way with nerve terminals of primary afferents to sensitize them and thereby trigger a cascade of events that increases the sensitivity of the nerves [23]. During inflamation, nerve terminals are re-distributed and the sensitivity of muscular and serosal layers is increased, as shown by experiments in animals [24]. One cell could play a main role in these events: The mastocyte. Degranulation of mastocytes induces changes in intestinal motor patterns in animals, through stimulation of afferent pathways since effects of degranulation are cancelled when animals have been treated by capsaicin, which destroys afferent nerves [25]. In similar experiments, it was shown that inflammatory sensitization of afferent neurons increased their response rate [26]. Although it is too early to conclude from these experiments in animals, one must point out that in a subgroup of patients with positive allergenic skin tests and IBS symptoms, a challenge with the antigen dramatically accelerated intestinal transit [27]. On the other hand, inflammation significantly increases perception of rectal distension in animals [28] and involves neuromediators, like bradykinin, which usually do not mediate perception from the gut [29].

Hypersensitivity can thus be triggered by a number of factors (fig. 1) which are themselves able to influence digestive motility. These effects combine to induce abdominal symptoms, especially abdominal pain in patients with functional bowel disorder.s The discovery of a specific causal mechanism for this hypersensitivity could thus be the basis for an adapted treatment of these disorders, but would also lead to the recognition of distinct pathophysiological entities among functional bowel disorders.

A role for viscero-visceral reflexes

The extensive study of visceral afferents has shed light on the role of viscero-visceral reflexes which link the activity of different segments of the digestive tract, sometimes quite distant from each other. Some reflexes result from the activation of nerve loops constituted by the axons of primary afferent neurons themselves, which directly act on muscle or mucosal cells (for review, see [30]). The motor reflexes may be inhibitory ascendant, like the recto-colonic reflex elicited by distension tests in animals [28] or the colo-gastric reflex [31] or they may be excitatory like the gastro-colonic reflex responsible for the colonic response to eating [32]. These reflexes are modulated by stress and are modulated by drugs affecting the processing of sensations by afferents, like fedotozine which inhibits the colo-gastric reflex triggered by distension [31] and the antagonists of serotonin 5-HT_3 receptors which inhibit the recto-colonic inhibitory reflex triggered by lower gut distension [28].

The reflexes are also observed in humans. Voluntary suppression of defecation slows gastric emptying in healthy subjects [33]. In IBS patients, intra-rectal injection of glycerol induces a composite recto-colonic reflex associating a relaxation of the left colon and the onset of several massive contractions [34]. These massive contractions coincide with abdominal cramps which the patients complain about. This test could be a model for pharmacological studies of abdominal pain in functional patients.

Other viscero-visceral reflexes lead to secretory or vasular responses, either through axon reflexes or through reflexes occurring at the level of pre-spinal ganglia, at the spinal level or even through long reflexes like vago-vagal reflexes. Sympathetic afferents are also involved in the processing of these reflexes to the spinal structures [35].

Beside the viscero-visceral reflexes, the study of digestive afferents has also characterized and quantified viscero-somatic reflexes. The number of contractions of abdominal striated muscles has been used to measure the intensity of painful sensations triggered by luminal distension of the gut in animals [28]. In man, the R III reflex, involving a peripheral nerve and a striated muscle is influenced by sensitization or summation of effects provoked by a painful distension of one segment of the gut [36]. These studies remain experimental at the moment, but they could be the basis for a more objective approach to measurements of visceral sensitivity, and thereby could lead to new diagnostic procedures of functional digestive disorders.

For the clinician, what is the current output?

The question is whether the concept of visceral hypersensitivity will bring new diagnostic tools and therapeutic means to the clinician in treating functional bowel disorders?

From the pathophysiological point of view, digestive hypersensitivity, mainly demonstrated by distension studies, seems to be common to the various syndromes clustered in functional digestive disorders, independently of the classical distinction between disorders attributed to the foregut, like non-cardiac chest pain or non-ulcer dyspepsia or to the lower gut, like IBS. Hypersensitivity may not even be limited to the segment of the gut classically regarded as the origin of symptoms [4]. Several factors influence the perception and nociceptive thresholds and can thus interfere with results of multicenter trials or with the clinical use of the distension test. The technical protocols for performing these tests must be clearly defined, before proposing them for large clinical studies.

Advances expected over the next few years in the understanding of visceral afferents function, and relationships between the immune systems, inflammatory processes and nvervous control of digestive functions, will certainly lead to the recognition of different diseases based on different pathophysiological mechanisms, but no more defined by clusters of symptoms. However, this scientific approach to functional bowel disorders is expected to face some difficulty with the multimodal patterns of these disorders and the presence of multiple causes for the disorder at the same time in one patient.

The nearest and most important result for the clinician regards the development of new medical treatments for the management of patients with functional digestive disorders. The presence of receptors for a large number of neuromediators on visceral afferents, as well as the demonstration that several of these receptors are involved in the processing of sensations originating from the abdomen indicates that drugs acting as agonists or antagonists on these receptors could have a therapeutic benefit for the management of abdominal pain related to functional bowel disorders. Among the classes of pharmacological agents currently in clinical development, 5-HT_3 antagonists of serotonin, the "x-setrons" have been shown to influence visceral perception by acting on afferent nerve pathways, but also by modifying the compliance of the digestive wall, i. e., its ability to adapt to the imposed distension [38, 39]. Fedotozine, an agonist of peripheral kappa opiate receptors, is able to increase the thresholds of visceral perception of colonic distension, up to normal level in patients with IBS and a characterized hypersensitivity to distension [16]. In both cases, these compounds have shown a clinical activity in multicenter trials involving IBS patients [39, 40]. Other agents are potential candidates but at the moment we only have results from animal studies: tachykinins, bradykinin, vasopressin and oxytocin.

Conclusion

The recognition of visceral hypersensitivity in patients with functional digestive disorders has led to a better understanding of the pathophysiology of these conditions. However, numerous questions remain open. Future studies need to determine the factors actually responsible for the onset of visceral hypersensitivity as well as the structural or functional abnormalities which explain it at the level of visceral afferents. They must also determine the neurotransmitters and the receptors involved. The track is certainly open for years, but some results of clinical importance are already available for the clinician. The efforts of standardization of the distension tests will allow the clinicians to set up multicenter trials, using distension tests to select patients to be included. Better knowledge of the relationship between results of distension tests and clinical evolution of the patients may be expected from the results. Finally, the recognition of pharmacological targets on nerve afferents has led over the last five years to the development of new therapeutic approaches to functional bowel disorders.

Our understanding of functional digestive disorders will certainly improve within the next years. Syndromes will be categorized into different conditions with specific pathophysiological mechanisms. The Rome criteria will certainly be revisited!

References

[1] Lasser, R. B., Bond, J. H., Levitt, M. D.: The role of intestinal gas in functional abdominal pain. N Engl J Med 1975, 293: 523–526.
[2] Ritchie, J.: Pain from distension of the pelvic colon by inflating a balloon in the irritable colon syndrome. Gut 1973 14: 125–132.
[3] Bradette, M., Delvaux, M., Staumont, G., Fioramonti, J., Bueno, L., Frexinos, J.: Evaluation of colonic sensory thresholds in IBS patients using a barostat: definition of optimal conditions and comparison with healthy subjects. Dig Dis Sci 1994, 39: 449–457.
[4] Francis, C. Y., Houghton, L. A., Whorwell, P. J., Morris, J., Bradbury, J.: Enhanced sensitivity of the whole gut in patients with irritable bowel syndrome. Gastroenterology 1995, 108: A 601 (abstract).
[5] Bradette, M., Pare, P., Douville, P., Morin, A.: Visceral perception in health and functional dyspepsia. Crossover study of gastric distension with placebo and domperidone. Dig Dis Sci 1991, 36: 52–58.
[6] Castell, D. D.: Esophageal chest pain. Am J Gastroenterol 1984, 79: 969–976.
[7] Coremans, G., Tack, J., Vantrappen, G., Janssens, J., Annese, V.: Is the irritable bowel really irritable? Ital J Gastroenterol 1991, 23 (suppl 1): 39–40.
[8] Lloyd, D. A., Borda, I. T.: Food induced heartburn: effect of osmolality. Gastroenterology 1981, 80: 740–741.
[9] Kellow, J. E., Eckersley, G. M., Jones, M. P.: Enhanced perception of physiological intestinal motility in the irritable bowel syndrome. Gastroenterology 1991, 101: 1621–1627.
[10] Norton, S., Rosenweig, A.: The supersensitive esophagus: a possible cause of atypical chest pain in young women. Gastroenterology 1987, 95: 1600 (abstract).
[11] Accarino, A. M., Azpiroz, F., Malagelada, J. R.: Selective dysfunction of mechanosensitive intestinal afferents in Irritable Bowel Syndrome. Gastroenterology 1995, 108: 636–643.
[12] Lembo, T., Munakata, J., Mertz, H., Niazi, N., Kodner, A., Nikas, V., Mayer, E. A.: Evidence for the hypersensitivity of lumbar splanchnic afferents in irritable bowel syndrome. Gastroenterology 1994, 107: 1686–1696.
[13] Silverman, D. H. S., Munakata, J. A., Hoh, C. K., Mandelkern, M. A., Phelps, M. E., Blahd, W., Mayer, E. A.: Regional cerebral activity in normal and pathologic perception of visceral pain: An O-15-Water PET study of healthy subjects and IBS patients. Gastroenterology 1996, 110: A 759 (abstract).
[14] Munakata, J. A., Silverman, D. H. S., Hoh, C. K., Mandelkern, M. A., Blahd, W., Mayer, E. A.: Rectosigmoid sensitization correlates with thalamic response to rectal pain: an O-15-water PET study of normal subjects and IBS patients. Gastroenterology 1996, 110: A 720 (abstract).
[15] Thompson, W. G., Creed, F., Drossman, D. A., Heaton, K. W., Mazzacca, G.: Functional bowel disorders and chronic functional pain. Gastroenterol Int 1992, 5: 75–91.
[16] Delvaux, M., Louvel, D., Scherre, B., Fraitag, B., Frexinos, J.: The k-agonist Fedotozine increases thresholds of first sensation and pain perception to colonic distension in patients with Irritable Bowel Syndrome. Gastroenterology 1995, 108: A 590 (abstract).
[17] Prior, A., Maxton, D. G., Whorwell, P. J.: Anorectal manometry in irritable bowel syndrome: differences between diarrhoea and constipation predoinant subjects. Gut 1990, 31: 458–462.
[18] Houghton, L.-A., Wych, J., Whorwell, P.: Acute diarrhea induces rectal sensitivity in women but not men. Gut 1995, 37: 270–273.
[19] Mertz, H., Nalibott, B., Munakata, J., Niazi, N., Mayer, E. A.: Altered rectal perception is a biological marker of patients with irritable bowel syndrome. Gastroenterology 1995, 109: 40–52.

[20] Whitehead, W. E., Crowell, M. D., Davidoff, A., Cheskin, L., Schuster, M. M.: Is sexual abuse associated with lower thresholds for pain due to balloon distension of the rectum? Gastroenterology 1994, 106: A 588 (abstract).
[21] Ford, M. J., Camilleri, M., Zinsmeister, A. R., Hanson, R. B.: Psychosensory modulation of colonic sensation in the human transverse and sigmoid colon. Gastroenterology 1995, 109: 1772–1780.
[22] Khan, I., Collins, S. M.: Is there an inflammatory basis for a subset of patients presenting with diarrhoea in the irritable bowel syndrome? Gastroenterology 1994, 106: A 523 (abstract).
[23] Sidall, P. J., Cousins, M. J.: Pain mechanisms and management: An update. Clin Exp Pharmacol Physiol 1995, 22: 679–688.
[24] Stead, R. H., Kosecka-Janiszewska, U., Oestreicher, A. B., Dixon, M. F., Bienenstock, J.: Remodellling of B-50 (GAP-43)- and NSE-immunoreactive mucosal nerves in the intestines of rats infected with Nippostrongylus Brasiliensis. J Neurosci 1991, 11: 3809–3821.
[25] Castex, N., Fioramonti, J., Fargeas, M. J., Buéno, L.: c-fos Expression in specific rat brain nuclei after intestinal anaphyllaxis: involvement of 5-HT 3 receptors and vagal afferent fibers. Brain Res 1995, 688: 149–160.
[26] Eastwood, C., Grundy, D.: Mast cell modulation of intestinal afferents. Gastroenterology 1996, 110: A 659 (abstract).
[27] Malatesta, M. G., Forlani, G.; Falcucci, G.; Ciccaglione, A. F., Castellano, A., Travaglini, N., Grossi, L., Marzio, L.: Mouth to caecum transit time is accelerated after oral food antigen in patients with irritable bowel syndrome. Gastroenterology 1996, 110: A 712 (abstract).
[28] Morteau, O., Eeckhout, C., Buéno, L.: Effect of the 5-HT 3 antagonists (granisetron and KC 9946) on viscerosensitive response to colorectal distension before and during experimental colitis in awake rats. Fundam Clin Pharmacol 1994, 8: 553–562.
[29] Julia, V., Mezzasalma, T., Buéno, L.: Influence of bradykinin in gastrointestinal disorders and visceral pain induced by acute or chronic inflammation in rats. Dig Dis Sci 1995, 40: 1913–1921.
[30] Grund, D., Scratcherd, T.: Sensory afferents from the gastrointestinal tract. In: Wood, J. D.(ed.), Handbook of Physiology, Section 6, Volume 1, American Physiological Society, Bethesda, 1989, 593–620.
[31] Gué, M., Junien, J. L., Buéno, L.: The kappa agonist fedotozine, modulates colonic distension-induced inhibition of gastric motility and emptying in dogs. Gastroenterology 1994, 107: 1327–1334.
[32] Frexinos, J., Buéno, L., Fioramonti, J.: Diurnal changes is myoelectrical spiking activity of the human colon. Gastroenterology 1985, 88: 1104–1110.
[33] Tjeerdsma, H. C., Smout, A. J. P., Akkermans, L. M. A.: Voluntary suppression of defecation delays gastric emptying. Dig Dis Sci 1983, 38: 832–836.
[34] Louvel, D., Delvaux, M., Staumont, G., Camman, F., Fioramonti, J., Buéno, L., Frexinos, J.: Intracolonic injection of glycerol: A model for abdominal pain in Irritable Bowel Syndrome. Gastroenterology 1996, 110: 351–361.
[35] Renehan, W. E., Xuego, Z., Beierwaltes, W. H., Foger, R.: Neurons in the dorsal motor nucleus of the vagus may integrate vagal and spinal information from the gastrointestinal tract. Am J Physiol 1995, 268: G 780–G 790.
[36] Bouhassira, D., Coffin, B., Chollet, R., Fraitag, B., Genève, J., Willer, J. C., Jian, R.: Effect of fedotozine on gastric nociception assessed by a reflexologic technique. Gastroenterology 1995, 108: A 576 (abstract).
[37] Prior, A., Read, N. W.: Reduction of rectal sensitivity and postprandial motility by granisetron, a 5-HT 3 receptor antagonist, in patients with irritable bowel syndrome. Aliment Pharmacol Ther 1993, 7: 175–180.

[38] Delvaux, M., Louvel, D., Campos-Oriola, R., Forster, E., Frexinjos, J.: Effect of alosetron on colonic sensitivity in patients with irritable bowel syndrome (IBS). Gastroenterology 1996, 110: A 655 (abstract).

[39] Dapoigny, M., Abitbol, J. L., Fraitag, B.: Efficacy of peripheral kappa agonist fedotozine versus placebo in treatment of irritable bowel syndrome. A multicenter dose-response study. Dig Dis Sci 1995, 40: 2244–2248.

[40] Bardhan, K., Bodemar, G., Geldof, H., Schutz, E., Snell, C., Darekar, B.: A double-blind, placebo-controlled study to evaluate the efficacy of alosetron in the treatment of irritable bowel syndrome (IBS). Gastroenterology 1996, 110: A 630 (abstract).

Efficacy of Duspatalin® 200 mg in patients with irritable bowel syndrome: Results of a descriptive study on various symptom subgroups

P. Guyot

Introduction

Irritable bowel syndrome (IBS) is a particularly frequent occurrence. A number of epidemiological studies have shown that this type of illness occurs in about 20% of the adult population of the western world and it is estimated that it is the reason for about half of the consultations with specialists in gastroenterology [1]. After any necessary elimination of an organic lesion of the alimentary tract, the diagnosis of IBs is essentially clinical. It is based on the combination of three cardinal symptoms which have been developing for at least three months, namely abdominal pain, disturbed bowel habits (diarrhea or constipation) and sensations of abdominal meteorism (IBS). Abdominal pain is the essential and unvoidable symptom for arriving at a positive diagnosis of IBS and it is this which usually makes the patients consult their physician. Depending on the degree of combination of these three symptoms, it is possible to classify the patients in a particular clinical form such as was proposed at a meeting of international experts [2]. The essentil significance of this classification takes into account the polymorphic and highly variable nature of IBS, a factor which is nearly always ignored in the therapeutic studies published in literature.

Among the various pharmacological substances used for treatment of IBS, mebeverine has proved its efficacy in these patients over many years by its predominant musculotropic spasmolytic action [3]. nlike certain other antispasmodics, mebeverine demonstrates anticholinergic activity. It therefore does not produce undesirable side effects such as dryness of the mouth, blurred vision or urinary retention. In earlier studies, the efficacy of mebeverine 200 mg was determined in a general population of patients suffering from IBS without taking these various symptom subgroups into account [3]. The purpose of this multicentre descriptive study was to determine the efficacy of mebeverine 200 mg (Duspatalin® 200) in relation to the combination of the symptoms. Five symptom groups were identified according to the bowel habits and the presence or absence of abdominal distension combined with abdominal pain (tab. 1).

The therapeutic efficacy of a compound is sometimes difficult to determine in an open study. To approach this problem, very strict efficacy criteria were de-

Table 1 Demographic characteristics of the population included in the trial

Parameters		
Age (years): Mean standard variation (min.-max.)	35.5±8.40	(18.2–52.6)
Sex		
Male	29.3%	(93)
Female	70.7%	(225)
Alimentary history		
Mdical	17.7%	(56)
Surgical	33.3%	(106)
Concomitant treatment		
Yes	56.9%	(181)
No	43.1%	(137)
Use of a laxative		
Yes	4.4%	(14)
Other symptoms on Day 0		
Dryness of the mouth	21.4%	(68)
Drowsiness	15.1%	(48)
Blurred vision	6.6%	(21
Urination difficulties	1.3%	(4)
Palpitations	17.9%	(57)
Pain (min.) Mean±standard variation (min.–max.)	64.8±17.6	(16–100)

fined *a priori* for judging the efficacy of mebeverine 200 mg. A patient was defined as being a responder if the abdominal pain disappeared or was considered to be mild for at least 70% of the study period and if the other criteria (frequency and consistency of the stools, abdominal distensions, defaecation abnormalities) were normalized or were of low intensity. The incidence of the responder character was then determined in each of the five predefined groups and its confidence range was calculated. These values were compared with a theoretical value of 20% placebo response.

Aims and principles

This trial was performed in patients known to have been diagnosed as having IBS.

Each patient included in the trial was "ranged" in a symptomatic form according to the customary predominance of the gastrointestinal symptoms (Group I pain, diarrhea and distension, Group II pain, constipation and distension, Group III pain and diarrhea, Group IV pain and constipation, Group V pain

Table 2 Number of patients per symptom group

Group	Symptoms	Number of patients
I	Pain, diarrhoea, distension	75
II	Pain, constipation, distension	111
III	Pain, diarrhoea	23
IV	Pain, constipation	22
V	Pain, distension	87
	Total	318

and distension, tab. 2). This classification in a symptomatic form or "symptomatic profile" is convenient, as it permits classification of the polymorphic character of the IBS. On the other hand, it does not permit comparison between symptomatic forms as it is not a random affectation hazardous to a group. The statistical analysis is consequently purely descriptive.

The definition of the efficacy criterion comprises two parts. The first is that of "responder patient", that is, a patient in whom the abdominal pain is of low intensity or absent for at least 70% of the time, the frequency of defaecations has normalized, the consistency of the stools has normalized and the abdominal distensions are of mild intensity or absent. The second is that of "responder group": The frequency of occurrence of the "responder" character is calculated for each group. The confidence range ($\alpha = 0.05$) of the frequency of occurrence of the "responder" character is then calculated.

The principal aim of this trial was to compare the frequency of occurrence of the "responder" character to the treatment in the study of the patients in each group with that of a qualified theoretical frequency of absence of therapeutic response (20% level taking account of the severity of the definition of "responder patient").

Methods and population studied

Methods

Non-comparative, descriptive, multicentre (anticipated 75 centres), phase IV trial, taking account of the number of patients to be included determined on the basis of the initial hypotheses.

Illness

The existence of IBS was defined by the Rome criteria [2]. The abdominal pain should furthermore be of an intensity equal to or greater than 2 (frequent and/or prolonged, difficult to relieve and interfering with many social activities).

Patients

To be included in this trial, each patient had to satisfy the following selection criteria:

- Age between 18 and 50 years, existence of IBS, written consent to take part in the trial. A morphological exploration of the colon within the last three years was necessary for patients over 40 years old.
- The pain had to be a manifestation of IBS and not an organic disease. The other restrictions to inclusion were represented on the one hand by the regulatory obligations and on the other hand by the contraindications and precautions for administration of the trial compound.

Study medication

- The study medication was given on Day 0 after verification of the selection criteria.
- The study medication was Duspatalin® 200, which is available as gelatin capsules each containing 200 mg coated microgranules of mebeverine.
- The dosage was that recommended in the package leaflet, i. e., one 200 mg capsule in the morning and one 200 mg capsule in the evening.
- Each patient had to take the treatment for eight weeks.
- The investigator checked that the patient was taking the treatment by counting the therapeutic units remaining whenever the patient reported for evaluation of the efficacy of the treatment.

Concomitant treatment

- The only other authorized drugs were liquid paraffin oil as laxative and/or aspirin as analgesic (in a maximum dose of 500 mg per day administered on fewr than five occasions throughout the trial). The name and dosage of the medication had to be noted on the record forms.
- The use of any other medication, especially antispasmodics and gastric or other intestinal drugs, was prohibited.

Evaluations

- The investigator evaluated the clinical state of the patient three times: During verification of the selection criteria and of the allocation of treatment, then after four weeks of treatment and after eight weeks.
- The patient evaluated the intensity of his/her pain daily on a four-point scale.

Monitoring

Monitoring was carried out by each investigator in accordance with Good Clinical Practice (GCP).

Principal criterion of efficacy

Comparison of the proportion of "responder" patients in each group with that of "non-responders".

Analysis of data

- Analysis of the efficacy was carried out as "intention to treat", that is, on the data of all the patients who had taken one therapeutic unit at least once and in whom at least one evaluation of the symptomatology had taken place.
- The missing data on a variable were replaced by the last known value of this variable.

The "responder" character was determined for all the included patients:

- At the final point or "final day" that this evaluation had taken place after eight weeks (the patient normally having completed the trial), or between Day 0 and eight weeks (the patient having prematurely stopped participating in the trial), or after eight weeks (evaluation delayed beyond the time limits) (fig. 1).
- After eight weeks (tolerance of two days around this date of evaluaton) (fig. 2).

At the points Week (W one to eight: development of the weekly mean intensity of the abdominal pain, based on the data collected by the patient on the self-assessment given to him/her on Day 0.

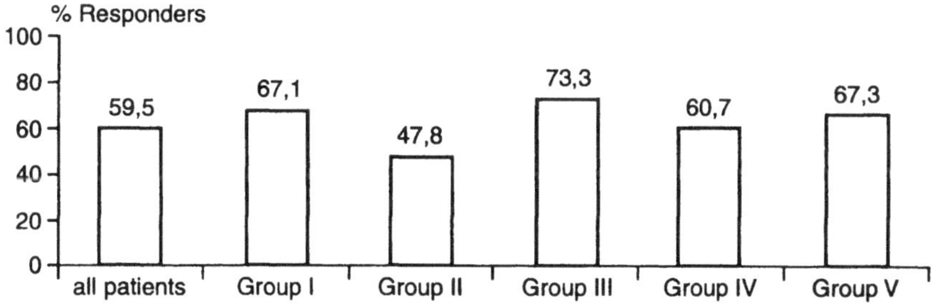

Fig. 1 Responders after 8 weeks treatment (n = 276).

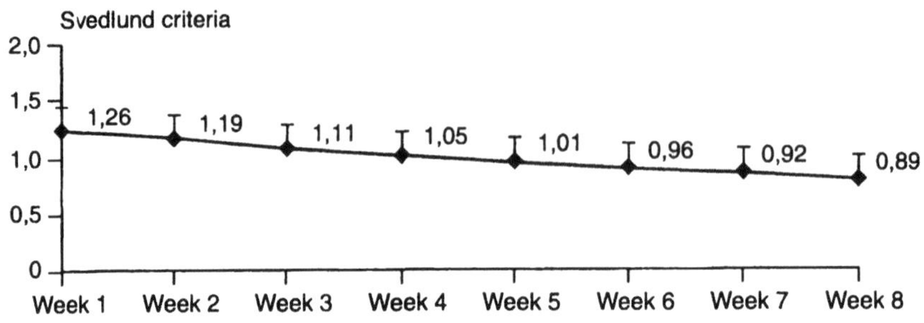

Fig. 2 Pain evaluation via self-assessment booklet of all 5 groups.

Results

The agreement of the CCPPRB (ethic committee) of Lyon was obtained in October 1994. The trial was performed from October 1994 to October 1995.

Monitoring of the patients was ensured by their visits to the centres, immediately followed by correspondence aimed at correcting incorrect data and filling in missing data.

Population included in the trial and stopping of treatment

- 318 patients were included in this trial by 60 general practitioners located throughout France (General Practitioners Research Association).
- Patients completed the eight weeks of treatment.
- The treatment was discontinued prematurely in a total of 42 patients, namely by the patients themselves in 29 cases or by the investigator (seven patients) or by a third party (three patients) or by mutual agreement between investigator and patient (three patients). There was either just one reason for stopping treatment in the individual cases (inclusion error in two cases, violation of the protocol in one case, occurrence of an undesirable (side) effect in five cases, absence of efficacy iin nine cases, disappearance of the symptoms before the normal term in two cases, "weariness" on the part of the patient in three cases), or a number of reasons (in 20 cases).

Deviation from the protocol

Two types of deviations can be described schematically and they very often occurred in combination with each other:

- Major deviations, relating to the intensity of the pain (in two cases) or to administration of unauthorised medicartion (in 17 cases).
- Minor deviations: 440.

Tolerance

The tolerance was excellent. Only 12 cases were seen to be related to the medication. Most of them are in relation to the IBS symptoms, e. g. constipation, diarrhea, nausea, gastralgia and flatulence (eight cases). In two cases dry mouth was described and in two a slight increase of the the body temperature. Only two of the 12 cases (constipation) were judged to be severe, the others were mild or moderate.

Discussion

The results of this study confirm that mebeverine 200 mg improves the symptoms of patients suffering from irritable bowel syndrom irrespective of the symptom profile considered (tab. 3).

The principal reason for which IBS patients consult their physician is abdominal pain which, due to its frequency, its chronic nature and the inconvenience that it causes directly interferes with the patient quality of life (daily life, relationships, etc.) [4]. Consideration of this criterion, which was the principal assessment criterion, showed that the proportion of patients responding to mebeverine (almost 60% after 8 weeks) was significantly greater than the theoretical level of inefficacy defined at the outset and was always found to be within the predetermined confidence limits. The poorest response was obtained in the group combining pain, abdominal distension and constipation. However, the results must be interpreted in relation to the study criteria, which did not permit concomitant treatment with laxatives, apart from liquid paraffin oil, which was in any case hardly ever effective. Clinical experience clearly shows that this type of patient nearly always needs treatment with an active laxative such as an osmotic laxative or fibre supplements in combination with antispasmodics.

Consideration of the other symptoms independently of the bowel evacuation disorders, showed that mebeverine significantly increased the frequency of defaecation and mormalized the consistency of the stools equally well in constipated patients and in those with diarrhea. This effect is explained by the regulatory action of mebeverine on the motility of the gastroitestinal tract [6]. Similarly, the other associated symptoms which are often ignored in therapeutic studies on IBS, such as urgent need to evacuate the bowels, sensation of incomplete rectal evacuation or difficulty in evacuating the bowels during strenuous defaecation, had completely disappeared in more than 80% of the patients, irrespective of the symptom group. These complaints to be sure are often acknowledged by the patients to be merely secondary complaints, but they nonetheless produce the need to find a cure.

Table 3 Development of symptoms

Parameters (all groups together)	Number of patients	Frequency %
Abdominal pain during the final 7 days		
None	121	38.05
Occasional	137	43.08
Frequent	5	16.98
Severe	6	1.89
Median	1	
Abdominal pain compared to the start		
disappeared	104	33.7
alleviated	138	44.7
unchanged	58	18.8
became worse	9	2.9
Weekly stool frequency (final week)		
m ± sd (n)	8.3±6.3 (318)	
Weekly stool consistency (final week)		
median(n)	0 (318)	
Difficulty in bowel evacuation		
Absent	241	75.8
Present	77	24.2
Sensation of incomplete evacuation		
Absent	222	69.8
Present	96	30.2
Sensation of urgent need to evacuate bowel		
Absent	252	79.2
Present	66	20.8
Distensions		
None	119	37.4
Occasional	131	41.2
Frequent	59	18.5
Continuous	9	2.8

The pathophysiological mechanisms involved in IBS are often numerous and complex [5]. Hypersensitivity to mechanical distension but also intestinal motility abnormalities have been widely demonstrated by numerous studies reported in the literature. By virtue of its musculotropic spasmolytic activity, mebeverine acts directly on the gastro-intestinal muscle cell, which is the terminal effector agent on which all these abnormalities are concentrated. A recent study has just shown that mebeverine, administered in a dose identical to that used in this study (200 mg × 2), was capable of correcting, upon the first dose, the intestinal motility abnormalities in IBS patients equally well in cases of diarrhea and in cases of constipation [6]. As there are many areas in which the intestinal motility and sensitivity can be checked and controlled, it is logical to propose a prolonged treatment (eight weeks) for correcting the abnormalities responsible here. It should be noted that the symptoms were improved as from the time of the mid-study visit (four weks) but that this improvement continued right up to the end of the observation period (eight weeks).

Conclusions

In conclusion, this therapeutic study performed in 318 patients confirms that mebeverine 200 mg is an effective and safe treatment for irritable bowel syndrome, irrespective of the patient subgroups. Mebeverine 200 mg causes the disappearance of not only the pain, but also of the other symptoms experienced by the patient and thus permits a general improvement in the patient's condition. This efficacy increases with time, thus justifying prolonged treatments in order to obtain a full effect.

References

[1] Bommelaer, G., Dapoigny, M.: Troubles fonctionnels intestinaux: définition, Epidémiologie. (Intestinal function disorders: definition, epidemiology). Progrès en Hépato-gastroentérologie, Vol. 11, Paris Editions Doin, 1955, 136–147.

[2] Thompson, W. G. and the Working Team for Functional Bowel Disorders: Functional bowel disorders and functional abdominal pain. In: Drossman, D. E. (ed.): The functional gastrointestinal disorders. Boston Little Brown Editions, 1994, 115–173.

[3] Berthelot, J. et al.: Etude contrôlée en double aveugle Duspatalin (mébévérine) contre placebo dans le traitement du colon irritable. (Controlled double-blind study on Duspatalin (mebeverine) versus placebo in the treatment of the irritable colon). Gazette Médicale de France 1981, 88: 2341–2343.

[4] Pauwels, A., Denis, P.: Troubles fonctionnels intestinaux: le patient face à ses symptômes (Intestinal function disorders: How can the patient deal with his symptoms?) Act Med Int – Gastroentérologie 1995, 9 (10) Supplement.

[5] Frexinos, J., Louvel, D., Delvaux, M.: Physiopathologie des troubles fonctionnels intestinaux (Physiopathology of intestinal function disorders) Progrès en Hépato-Gastroentérologie, Vol. 11, Paris Editions Doion, 1966, 124–136.

[6] Evans, P. R., Bak, Y. T., Kellow, J. E.: Mebeverine alters small bowel motility in irritable bowel syndrome. Aliment Pharmacol Ther 1996, 10: 787–793.

Clinical experience with mebeverine 200 mg

C. P. Fletcher

"Nowhere is the art of medicine more necessary than in the diagnosis and treatment of irritable bowel syndrome (IBS). Patients may suffer greatly, both physically and mentally, and doctors should view these people as presenting a real challenge to their diagnostic acumen and therapeutic skills" [1].

Introduction

Irritable bowel syndrome (IBS) is characterized by abdominal pain and alteration in bowel habit. The disordered bowel habit may consist of either constipation or diarrhoea or an alteration of the two. It is an extremely common disorder accounting for up to half of all cases seen by gastroenterologists [2, 3].

Mebeverine is a spasmolytic agent whose efficacy in IBS appears to be mediated via an effect on intracellular calcium concentrations [4]. By reducing the availability of free calcium in smooth muscle cells of the colon wall, mebeverine reduces the propensity of the gut to contract. This is thought to be the basis of the clinical efficacy of mebeverine [5].

For many years the licensed dose of mebeverine was 135 mg t. d. s (three times a day). This is a well established treatment regimen and has been demonstrated to have excellent efficacy and safety profiles [6, 7].

Due to the pharmacokinetic profile of mebeverine a new dosage form was developed: Mebeverine slow release microgranules 200 mg in capsules. Compared to a daily dosage of 400 mg the 200 mg b. d. (twice a day) should have equal efficacy to 135 mg t. d. s. This new formulation would also have the potential of increasing patient compliance over that of the three times daily dose.

Previous work by Inauen W. and Halter F., suggests that a regimen of 200 mg b. d. has a similar level of efficacy and adverse events to 135 mg t. d. s. [8].

Key previous mebeverine 200 mg studies

Inauen and Halter, 1994 [8]

This was the first study to compare the clinical efficacy, safety and tolerance of mebeverine slow release (200 mg) vs mebeverine 135 mg tablets in patients with IBS.

It was an open prospective parallel group three-center study in which 54 patients with irritable bowel syndrome were randomized to receive oral mebeverine slow release 200 mg twice daily (n = 26) or mebeverine tablets 135 mg three times daily (n = 28) for three weeks.

The assessments were performed at baseline and after one and three weeks of treatment. These included symptom severity, need for concomitant therapy and investigator's global impression of efficacy.

Symptoms explored using a four-point scale: eight gastrointestinal symptoms: abdominal pain, distension, constipation, diarrhoea, alternating constipation/diarrhea, appetite, nausea, vomiting and three non-gastrointestinal symptoms: anxiety, depression, tiredness.

The analysis of data did not show any significant difference in relative efficacy between the two groups with regard to the symptom scores.

Good or excellent efficacy was seen in 79% of mebeverine 135 mg patients, and 92% of mebeverine 200 mg patients. The investigator's global impression of efficacy after treatment also did not demonstrate a significant difference between the two treatment groups. No adverse events were reported. Both the tablet and retard formulations were safe and well tolerated. Systolic/diastolic blood pressures showed no change over time or differences between products.

Van Outryve et al., 1995 [9]

This was a double-blind crossover comparison study of the safety and efficacy of mebeverine slow release 200 mg capsules vs 135 mg tablets both with double dosages in the treatment of IBS.

Two centers in Belgium enrolled 72 IBS outpatients in this double-blind double-dummy study. Patients with a confirmed diagnosis of IBS (using the diagnostic scale of Kruis, and scores over 44 to include patients in the study), were given a one-week placebo baseline period and then randomized to six weeks of either 135 mg × 2 t. d. s. or 200 mg × 2 b. d. (this constitutes a double dose) in a crossover design.

Efficacy, tolerance and compliance were assessed before and after placebo week, and after three, six, nine and 12 weeks of active treatment. Symptom scores (intensity – five point scale, frequency – four point scale) of the different IBS symptoms after three weeks of treatment were considered:

- abdominal pain, bloating, flatulence, constipation, diarrhoea, alternating stool pattern.

Both treatments had equivalent efficacy, safety and compliance. There were no significant differences between treatments.

Both treatments were effective, e. g.:

- Patient/investigator evaluation after six weeks showed that both treatment forms (mebeverine plain and mebeverine 200 mg) were regarded as "effective" or "very effective" by > 80% of both groups.
- After three weeks of first treatment, disease score rated "light" in 73% patients in both treatment groups.
- After six weeks of first treatment period 33% patients were symptom free with mebeverine 135 mg and 18% with mebeverine 200 mg. During second treatment period 40% were symptom free in both groups.

Minor adverse events were recorded only, and judged to be unrelated to the study medications, although a double dosage was used.

Aims of the new 200 mg mebeverine study

The primary aim of the study was to show that mebeverine 200 mg b. d. has equivalent efficacy to mebeverine 135 mg t. d. s. in the treatment of abdominal pain in IBS assessed by VAS (Visual Analogue Scale).

The secondary aims were to investigate the safety of both formulations, and to evaluate physician's and patients' assessment of both formulations.

Study design

The study had a prospectively randomized double-blind, double-dummy design and was conducted over a period of one year between 1995–1996.

It was a multicenter study conducted by general practitioners in 22 United Kingdom practices. The original design required 270 patients to be recruited, with the aim of obtaining at least 184 patients with evaluable Case Record Forms. The study recruitment was terminated at 213 patients, because of a lower than anticipated dropout rate.

IBS was diagnosed to the Rome criteria, i. e., for at least three months abdominal pain and three or more additional IBS symptoms [10].

Patients who satisfied the inclusion/exclusion criteria had the severity of their IBS symptoms assessed and were then allocated to a regimen of either mebeverine 135 mg t. d. s. or 200 mg b. d. in a double-blind fashion for a eight weeks treatment period.

The assessments were repeated at four and eight weeks, after the patients commenced the study, at which point the study was completed.

Study procedures and assessments

The patients visited the physician on entering the study (Visit One), and at four and eight weeks after the start of the study (Visits Two and Three respectively).

For the assessments a Visual Analogue Scale (VAS) was administered on visits One to Three inclusive. They were completed by placing a single vertical mark on a 10 cm line at a point. VAS scales were used for maximum pain intensity during previous week, average pain intensity, present pain intensity and frequency of pain. Global VAS and "responders" were calculated from these VAS scales for the different visits by an algorithm.

Safety was assessed by the recording of adverse events and by the measurement of biochemistry, haematology and urinalysis.

The secondary efficacy variables were rated on a five-point scale: patients global assessment of therapeutic response, physician's global assessment of therapeutic response and physician's global impression of patient symptoms.

Efficacy

Of the 92 patients in each treatment group, 65 (71%) in the mebeverine 135 mg t. d. s. group and 64 (70%) in the mebeverine 200 mg b. d. group, were classified as "responders" (fig. 1). The difference between treatments in the percentage of responders is 1.5% with a 95% confidence interval of −12.8% to 15.8%. There was no statistically significant difference between treatment groups ($p = 0.84$).

This agrees with typical efficacy response rates seen with mebeverine in previous studies of around 75%.

The *Patients Assessment* of their response to therapy after four and eight weeks treatment, indicate no difference between treatments in the percentage of patients slightly/moderately/greatly improved. After four weeks, 80% of patients in the mebeverine 135 mg t. d. s. group were slightly/moderately/greatly improved compared to 76% in the mebeverine 200 mg b. d. group, with there being no difference between treatments ($p = 0.38$) (fig. 2).

After eight weeks 75% of patients in the mebeverine 135 mg t. d. s. group were slightly/moderately/greatly improved compared to 81% in the mebeverine 200 mg b. d. group, with there being no difference between treatments ($p = 0.47$) (fig. 2).

The *Physician's Assessment* of the clinical global impression of the disease symptoms are as shown in figure 3.

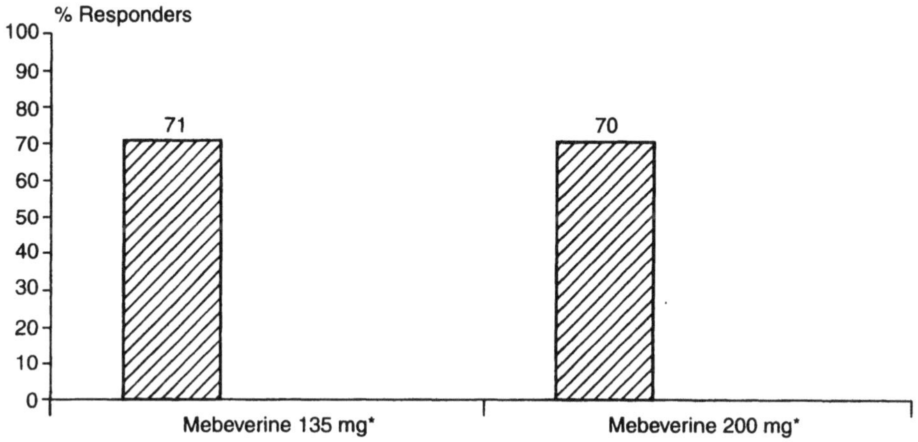

Fig. 1 Patient's assessment of ≥50% reduction of abdominal pain after 8 weeks treatment. *No difference between treatments in the percentage of "responders" ($p = 0.87$)

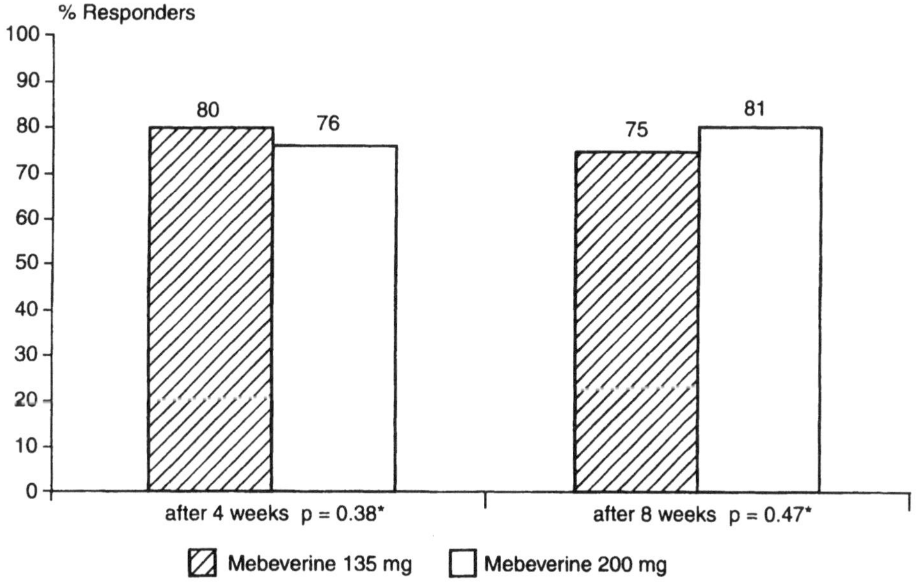

Fig. 2 Patient's assessment of secondary variables: global impression of symptom reduction and therapeutic response
* no difference between treatments

The Physician's Assessment of the clinical global evaluation of therapeutic response was between 79% – 84%, which is an excellent result for both preparations (fig. 4).

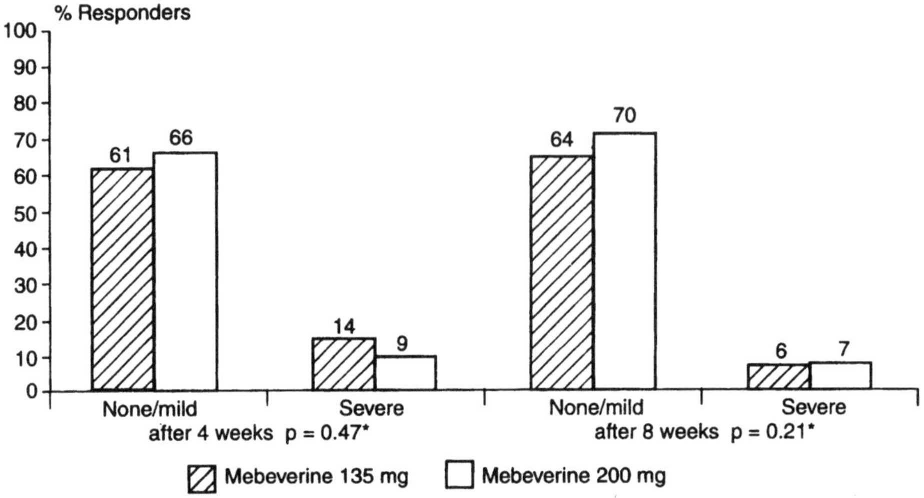

Fig. 3 Physician's assessment of symptoms (none, mild/severe)
* no difference between treatments

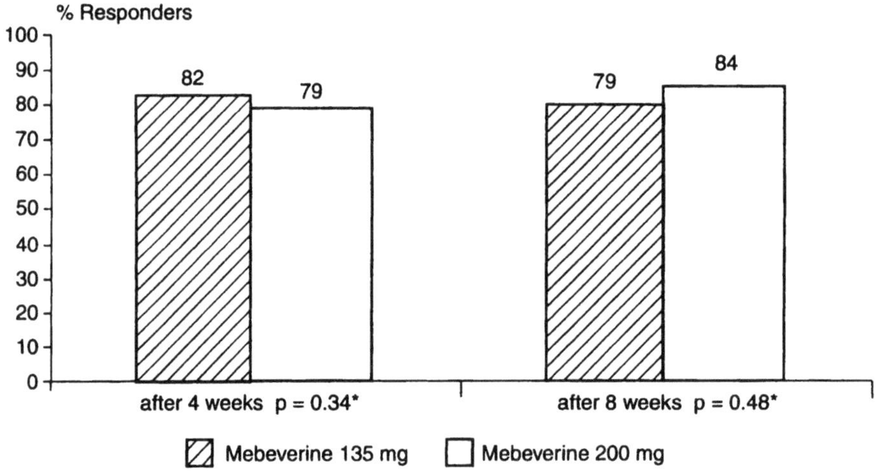

Fig. 4 Physician's assessment of response
* no difference between treatments

Safety

At least one adverse event was reported by 62% of patients in the mebeverine 135 mg t. d. s. group, and by 59% of patients in the mebeverine 200 mg b. d. group.

The most frequently reported adverse event was abdominal pain, reported by 9% of patients in the mebeverine 135 mg t. d. s. group and by 15% of patients in the mebeverine 200 mg b. d. group. Headache, nausea flatulence and diarrhoea were also relatively frequently, reported in both treatment groups.

Six serious adverse events were reported in total (pregnancy, bloody diarrhea in ulcerative colitis, elective surgery due to different reasons), but none was judged to be drug related.

Discussion

The primary aim of this double blind, multicentre study was to demonstrate equivalent efficacy of the new slow release formulation mebeverine 200 mg capsule b.d. versus the mebeverine 135 mg tablet t.d.s. This primary objective was achieved after four weeks and eight weeks treatment. The frequency of adverse events was comparable between the two formulations, and both demonstrated an excellent safety profile. The percentage of responders calculated from the global assessment via the VAS-scales are 71% for mebeverine 135 mg and 70% for mebeverine 200 mg, which is close to the values known from other mebeverine studies.

Another interesting aspect of this study was to see whether the mebeverine efficacy data known from a number of clinical IBS studies in the past [6, 7] differed by using very rigid IBS criteria (abdominal pain for at least three months and three or more IBS symptoms [10]), strict exclusion criteria and an up-to-date design for the evaluation of IBS symptoms (four different VAS scales) [11]. The data with mebeverine, however, is in general as good as with "old" study designs. There were no problems conducting this type of IBS study in General Practice.

In about 60% of the IBS patients at least one adverse event was seen in both treatment groups. The figures seem to be higher than in other studies [8, 9], but most of these adverse events (abdominal pain, nausea, flatulence, diarrhoea) are closely related to IBS which makes it difficult to differentiate between an adverse event and a symptom due to the disease.

Conclusion

In this study, mebeverine 200 mg b. d. was shown to have equivalent efficacy to mebeverine 135 mg t. d. s. and comparable safety.

The degree of symptom improvement was in agreement with previous studies of mebeverine.

References

[1] Burns, D. G.: The irritable bowel syndrome – a study from private practice. SA Medical Journal 1985, 68: 397–401.

[2] Manning, A. P., Thompson, W. G., Heaton, K. W., Morris, A. F.: Towards positive diagnosis of the irritable bowel. Br Med J 1978, 2: 653–654.

[3] Harvey, R. F., Salih, S. Y., Read, A. E.: Organic and functional disorders in 2000 gastroenterology outpatients. The Lancet 19823, ii: 632–634.

[4] Den Hertog, A., Van den Akker, J.: Modification of α_1-receptor-operated channels by mebeverine in smooth muscle cells of guinea-pig taenia caeci Eur J Pharmacol 1987, 138: 367–374.

[5] Den Hertog, A., Van den Akker, J.: The action of mebeverine and metabolites on mammalian non-myelinated nerve fibres. Eur J Pharmacol 1987, 139: 353–355.

[6] Pace, F., Coremans, G., Dapoigny, M., Müller-Lissner, S. A., Smout, A., Stockbrügger, R. W., Whorwell, P. J.: Therapy of irritable bowel syndrome – An overview. Digestion 1995, 56: 433–442.

[7] Poynard, T., Naveau, S., Mory, B., Chaput, J. C.: Meteaanalysis of smooth muscle relaxants in the treatment of irritable bowel syndrome. Aliment Pharmacol Ther 1994, 8: 499–510.

[8] Inauen, W., Halter, F.: Clinical efficacy, safety and tolerance of mebeverine slow release (200 mg) versus mebeverine tablets in patients with irritable bowel syndrome. Drug Invest 1994, 8: 234–240.

[9] Van Outryve, M., Mayeur, S., Meeus, M. A., Rosillon, D., Hendrickx, B., Ceuppens, M.: A double-blind crossover comparison study of the safety and efficacy of mebeverine with mebeverine sustained release in the treatment of irritable bowel syndrome. Journal of Clinical Pharmacy and Therapeutics 1995, 20: 277–282.

[10] Drossman, D. A., Thompsen, W. G., Talley, N. J., Funch-Jensen, P., Janssens, J., Whitehead, W. E.: Identification of sub-groups of functional gastrointestinal disorders. Gastroenterol Int 1990, 3: 159–172.

[11] Talley, N. J., Nyren, O., Drossman, D. A., Heaton, K. W., Veldhuiyzen van Zanten, S. J. O., Koch, M. M., Ransohoff, D. F.: The irritable bowel syndrome: Toward optimal design to controlled treatment trials. Gastroenterol Int 1993, 6: 189–211.

Bei Fragen zur Produktsicherheit wenden Sie sich bitte an:
If you have any questions regarding product safety,
please contact:

Walter de Gruyter GmbH
Genthiner Straße 13
10785 Berlin
productsafety@degruyterbrill.com